SOMATIC EXERCISES FOR BACK PAIN RELIEF

The Practical and Effective Exercises For Back Pain Relief, Improved Joint Health, Mobility, Balance, Flexibility, and Overall Well-being

LAURA C. AUSTIN

Copyright Page

TABLE OF
CONTENTS

INTRODUCTION

In the realm of chronic discomfort, back pain stands as a formidable adversary, affecting millions worldwide and disrupting daily routines with persistent discomfort. Traditional approaches often target symptoms rather than addressing the underlying causes, leading to temporary relief at best. However, amidst this challenge, somatic exercises emerge as a beacon of hope, offering a holistic pathway to alleviate back pain by reawakening the body's innate wisdom and self-healing mechanisms.

Somatic exercises, rooted in the principles of sensory motor learning, delve beyond the surface of muscles and joints, delving into the intricate relationship between the body and mind. At their core lies the concept of Sensory Motor Amnesia (SMA), wherein habitual patterns of tension become ingrained, leading to restricted movement and discomfort. Through gentle, mindful movements and the art of pandiculation, somatic exercises aim to unravel these patterns, restoring fluidity and freedom to the body.

This guide is a testament to the transformative power of somatic exercises in the realm of back pain relief. From understanding the mind-body connection to delving into essential exercises and addressing common queries, this guide aims to empower individuals on their journey towards reclaiming vitality and harmony within their bodies.

As we embark on this exploration of somatic exercises for back pain relief, let us open our hearts and minds to the profound wisdom inherent within our bodies, ready to embrace the transformative journey ahead.

WHAT ARE SOMATIC EXERCISES

Somatic exercise is all about tuning into your body's sensations and movements. It's like learning to speak the language of your muscles. By practicing somatic exercises, you become more aware of areas where you hold tension or move inefficiently. Through gentle movements and focused attention, you can release that tension and improve how your body feels and functions.

Think of it as reprogramming your body's software. You're teaching your brain to communicate better with your muscles, so they can relax when they're supposed to and engage when they're needed. This can lead to better posture, smoother movement, and reduced aches and pains.

Somatic exercises can be done lying down, sitting, or standing, and they often involve slow, deliberate movements combined with mindful breathing. The goal is to bring attention to areas of tension, gently release it, and gradually improve your overall body awareness and control. It's like giving yourself a massage from the inside out!

PRINCIPLES OF SOMATIC EXERCISES

Somatic exercises are a form of movement therapy that focuses on increasing body awareness, releasing muscular tension, and improving overall movement patterns. A field that explores the mind-body connection and emphasizes the role of sensory awareness in movement and posture.

- **SENSORY AWARENESS:** Somatic exercises begin with developing awareness of bodily sensations, such as muscle tension, joint mobility, and breathing patterns. By paying attention to these sensations, individuals can identify areas of tension or restriction in their bodies.

- **PANDICULATION:** Pandiculation is a fundamental concept in somatic exercises. It involves a three-step process of contracting a muscle, slowly releasing the contraction, and then allowing the muscle to relax fully. This process helps to reset the resting length of the muscle and release chronic tension.

- **MIND-BODY CONNECTION:** is a two-way relationship where the mind influences the body, and the body influences the mind. Somatic exercises emphasize the connection between the mind and body. By consciously engaging with movement and focusing on sensations, individuals can improve their ability to control and coordinate their movements.

- Functional Movement Patterns: Somatic exercises often focus on improving functional movement patterns that are relevant to everyday activities. By practicing movements such as reaching, bending, and twisting, individuals can improve their overall movement efficiency and reduce the risk of injury.

HOW SOMATIC EXERCISES DIFFER FROM TRADITIONAL APPROACHES TO BACK PAIN RELIEF

Somatic exercises differ from traditional approaches to back pain relief in several ways.

- **Focus on Sensory-Motor Learning**: Somatic exercises emphasize sensory-motor learning, which involves re-educating the nervous system to release muscle tension and restore proper movement patterns. Traditional approaches often focus on passive treatments like medication, injections, or surgeries, which may not address the underlying neuromuscular imbalances contributing to the pain.

- **Active Participation**: Somatic exercises require active participation from the individual experiencing back pain. Instead of relying solely on external interventions (such as chiropractic adjustments or massages), somatic exercises empower individuals to become actively involved in their own healing process through mindful movement and self-awareness.

- **Holistic Approach:** Somatic exercises take a holistic approach to back pain relief, considering the interconnectedness of the body and mind. These exercises not only address physical tension but also explore the psychological and emotional factors that may contribute to chronic pain. Traditional approaches often focus solely on the physical symptoms without addressing the broader context of the individual's well-being.

- **Long-Term Solutions:** Somatic exercises aim to provide long-term solutions by addressing the root causes of back pain rather than merely alleviating symptoms temporarily. By teaching individuals to release chronic muscle tension and improve movement patterns, somatic exercises promote lasting changes that can help prevent future episodes of pain. In contrast, traditional approaches may offer short-term relief but fail to address the underlying issues, leading to recurring or persistent pain.

BENEFITS OF SOMATIC EXERCISES
FOR BACK PAIN

Somatic exercises is highly beneficial for managing back pain, offering a holistic approach that addresses both physical and mental aspects of discomfort. Here are some benefits:

- **Improved Body Awareness**: Somatic exercises focus on increasing awareness of bodily sensations and movements, helping individuals recognize and release tension or stress stored in muscles contributing to back pain.

- **Muscle Relaxation:** Somatic exercises can alleviate muscle tension and tightness that often contribute to back pain by promoting conscious relaxation of specific muscle groups.

- **Enhanced Flexibility and Mobility:** Regular practice of somatic exercises can improve flexibility and mobility in the spine and surrounding muscles, reducing stiffness and discomfort.

- **Postural Correction:** Somatic exercises emphasize proper alignment and posture, which can help lessen strain on the back and prevent future pain by promoting healthier movement patterns.
- **Stress Reduction**: Engaging in somatic exercises promotes relaxation and reduces stress levels, which can indirectly relieve back pain exacerbated by tension or anxiety.

- **Non-Invasive Approach**: Somatic exercises offer a non-invasive, drug-free alternative for managing back pain, making them suitable for individuals seeking natural methods of pain relief.
- **Long-Term Relief**: Unlike temporary solutions that only address symptoms, somatic exercises target underlying issues contributing to back pain, offering the potential for long-term relief and prevention of recurring discomfort of the pain.

- **Overall Well-being**: Beyond alleviating back pain, somatic exercises promote overall physical and mental well-being by fostering relaxation, mindfulness, and a deeper connection with one's body.

ESSENTIAL TIPS FOR EFFECTIVE EXERCISE

- **Start Slowly:** Begin with gentle exercises and gradually increase intensity and duration over time to avoid exacerbating pain or causing injury.

- **Focus on Core Strength:** Strengthening the core muscles, including the abdominal and back muscles, can provide support to the spine and improve posture, reducing strain on the back.

- **Incorporate Stretching:** Include stretching exercises to improve flexibility, alleviate muscle tightness, and enhance range of motion in the spine and surrounding muscles.

- **Mindful Movement:** Practice exercises mindfully, paying attention to proper form, alignment, and breathing techniques to avoid unnecessary strain on the back.

- **Listen to Your Body:** Pay attention to your body's signals and adjust exercises as needed to avoid overexertion or discomfort.

- **Stay Active:** Incorporate regular physical activity into your routine, including low-impact exercises like walking, swimming, or cycling

- **Balance Strength and Flexibility:** Aim for a balance between strengthening and stretching exercises to support a healthy spine, prevent imbalances, and reduce the risk of injury.

- **Stay Consistent:** Consistency is key to experiencing the benefits of exercise for back pain relief. Aim for regular, ongoing exercise to maintain strength, flexibility, and overall back health.

- **Patience and Persistence:** Be patient with your progress and stay persistent in your efforts to alleviate back pain through exercise. It may take time to see significant improvements, but consistent effort can lead to long-term relief and improved quality of life.

CHILD'S POSE

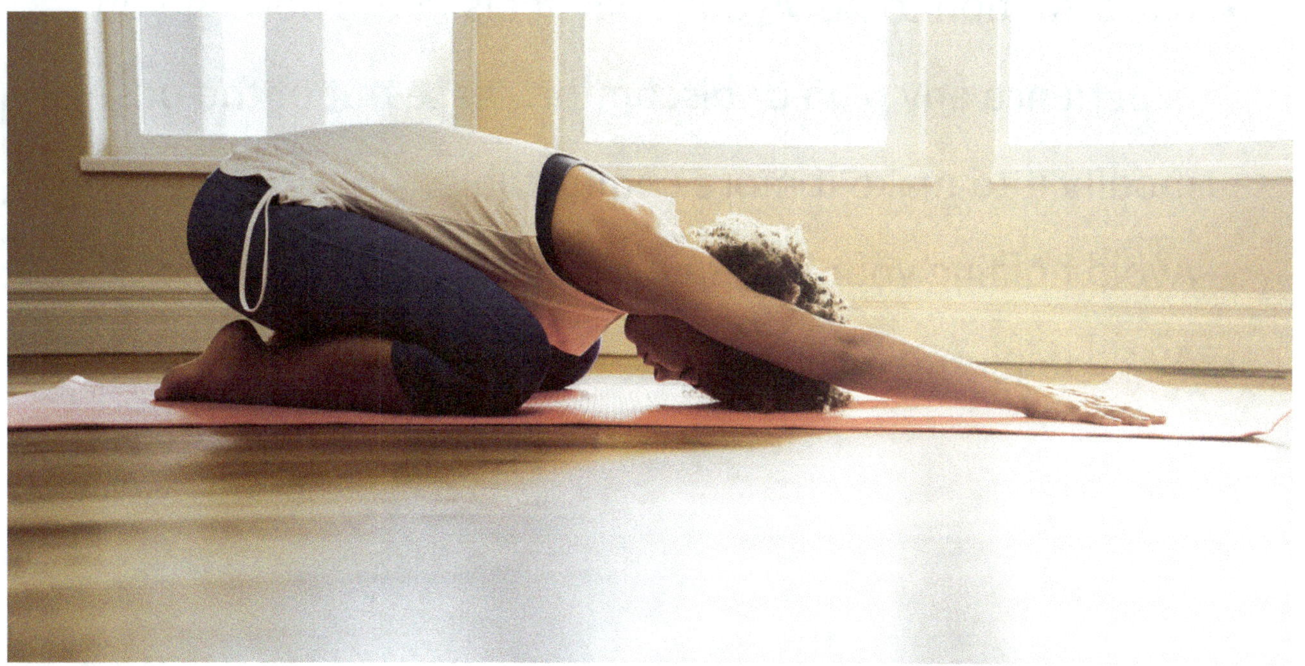

INSTRUCTIONS

- Begin by assuming a tabletop position, with your hands and knees on the ground.

- Release the tops of your feet to the floor and bring your knees wider than your hips, big toes touching.

- Gradually descend your hips toward your heels.

- Walk your hands forward and rest your head on the floor or a prop.

- Take several deep breaths, focusing on filling your belly and chest.

- Carefully return to the tabletop position.

SAFETY TIPS

- Pay attention to how your body feels in the pose. If you experience any pain or discomfort, ease out of the pose or modify it to make it more comfortable.
- Avoid holding your breath.
- Avoid if injured or pregnant

PELVIC TILTS

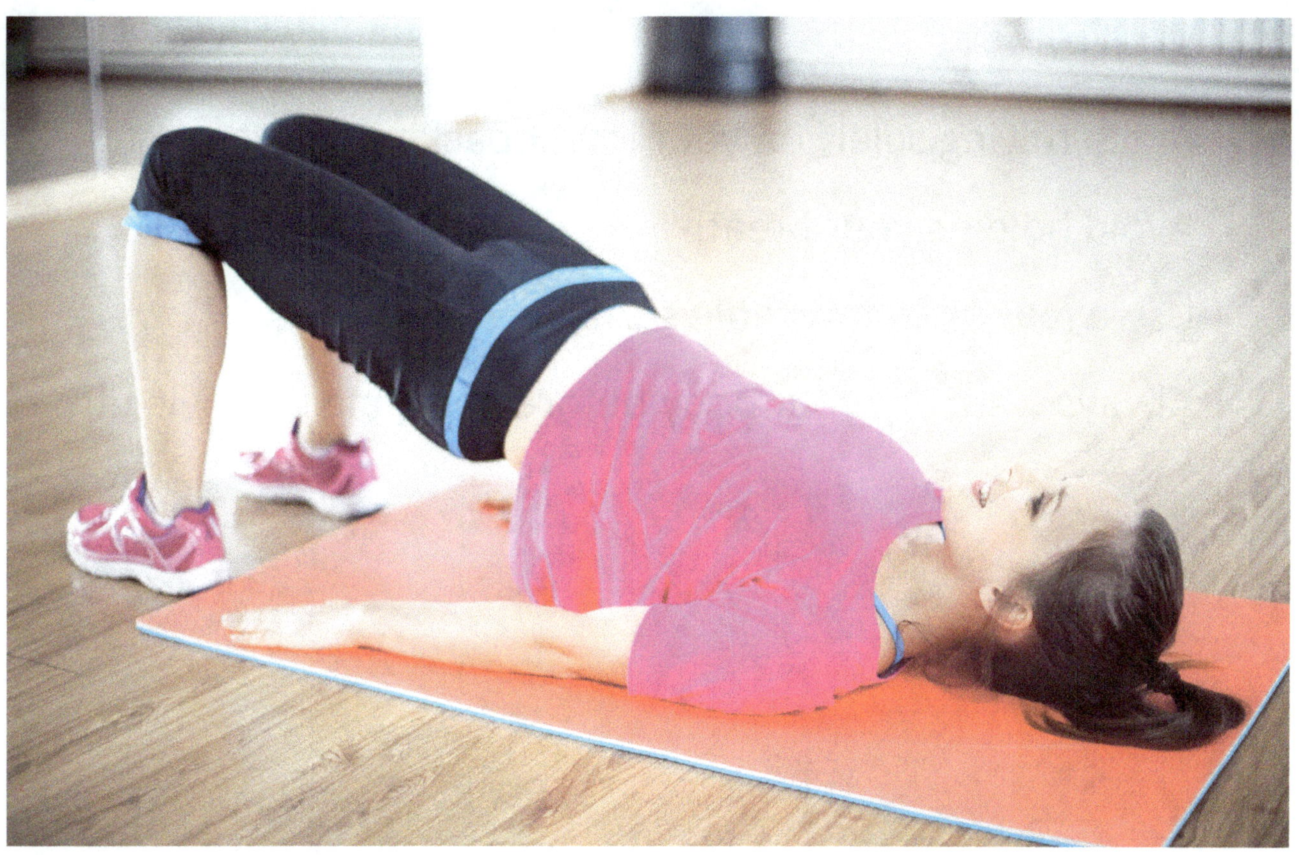

INSTRUCTIONS

- Start by lying on your back with your knees bent.

- Breathe in, and as you exhale, lift your pelvis upward.

- Inhale again to return to the starting position.

- Repeat this movement for 10-15 repetitions.

SAFETY TIPS

- Pay attention to your body alignment throughout the exercise.

- Avoid relying solely on your lower back for movement.

- Avoid holding your breath

- Use a mat or comfortable surface

- Always warm up your body before engaging in pelvic tilts.

SEATED FORWARD BEND

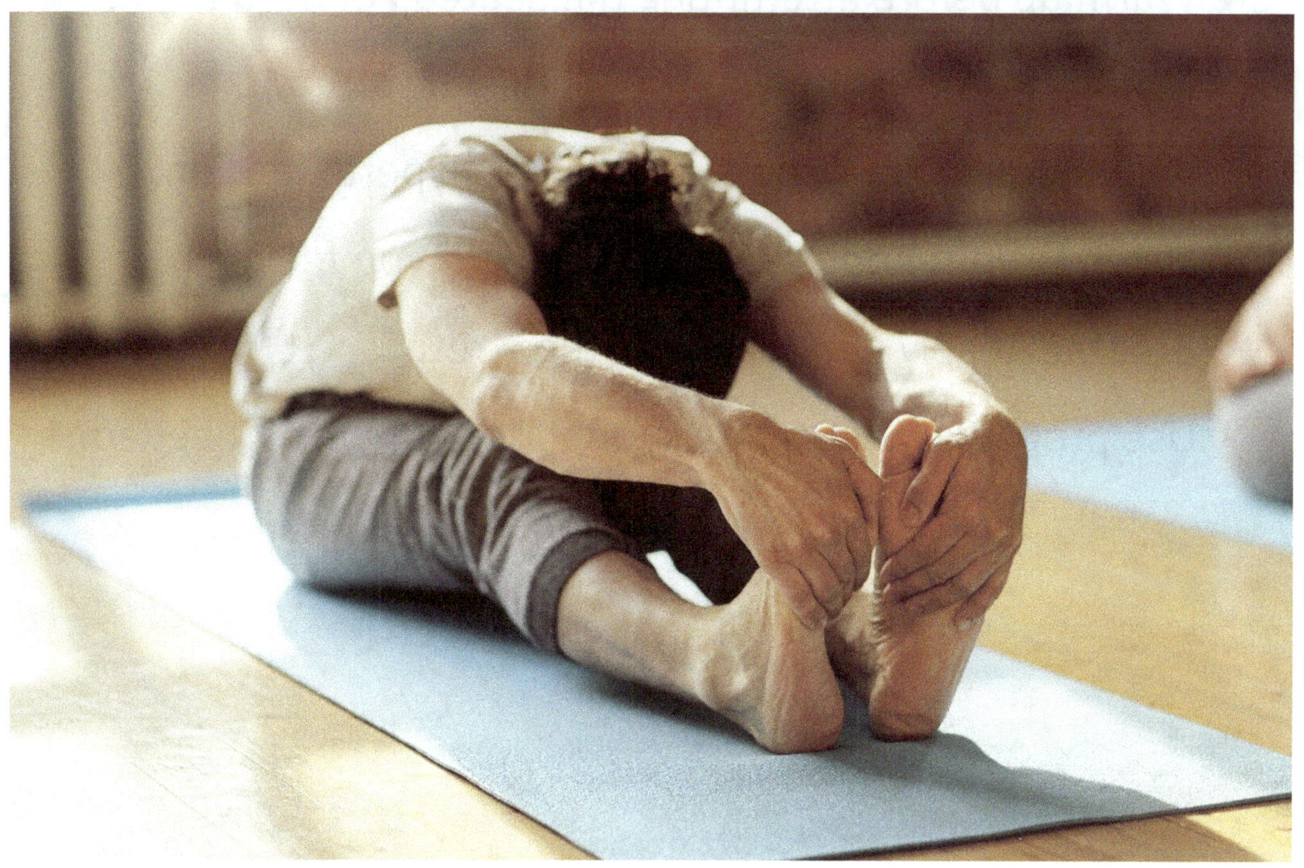

INSTRUCTIONS

- Begin by sitting with legs stretched out in front.

- Straighten your spine and elevate your chest.

- Lean forward from the hips, extending your hands towards your feet.

- Hold this position for 30 seconds to one minute.

- As you inhale, lift your torso back up.

SAFETY TIPS

- Warm up before attempting the Seated Forward Bend.

- Maintain a straight back throughout the stretch.

- Avoid locking your knees to prevent hyperextension.

- Listen to your body's signal and stop if you feel pain.

- Breathe deeply and relax into the stretch.

- Use props like a yoga block for added support if needed.

KNEE-TO-CHEST STRETCH

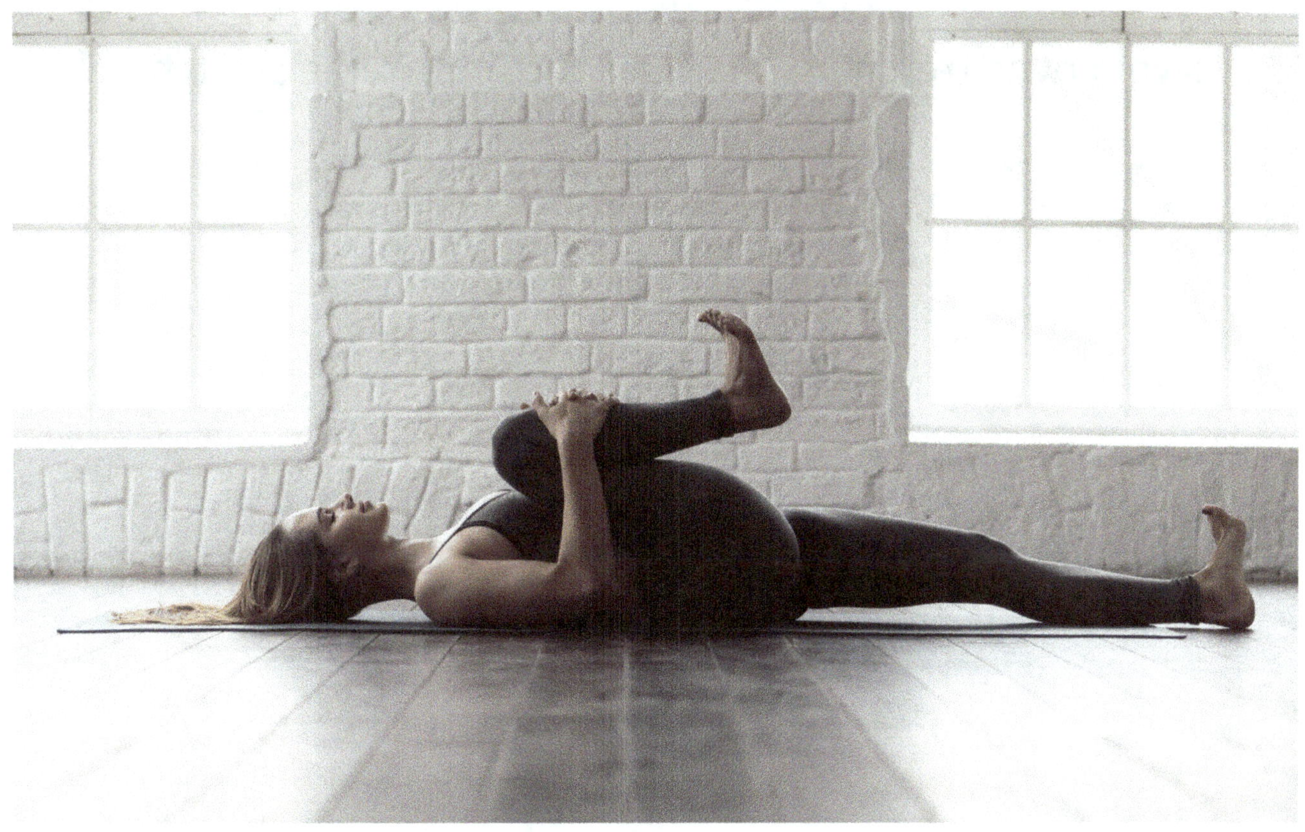

INSTRUCTIONS

- Start by lying on your back with your legs stretched out.

- Bring one knee towards your chest, holding it with both hands.

- Maintain this position for 15-30 seconds, experiencing a mild stretch.

- Then, switch to the other knee and repeat the process.

SAFETY TIPS

- Perform on a firm surface.

- Avoid overstretching; maintain a comfortable stretch.

CAT-COW STRETCH

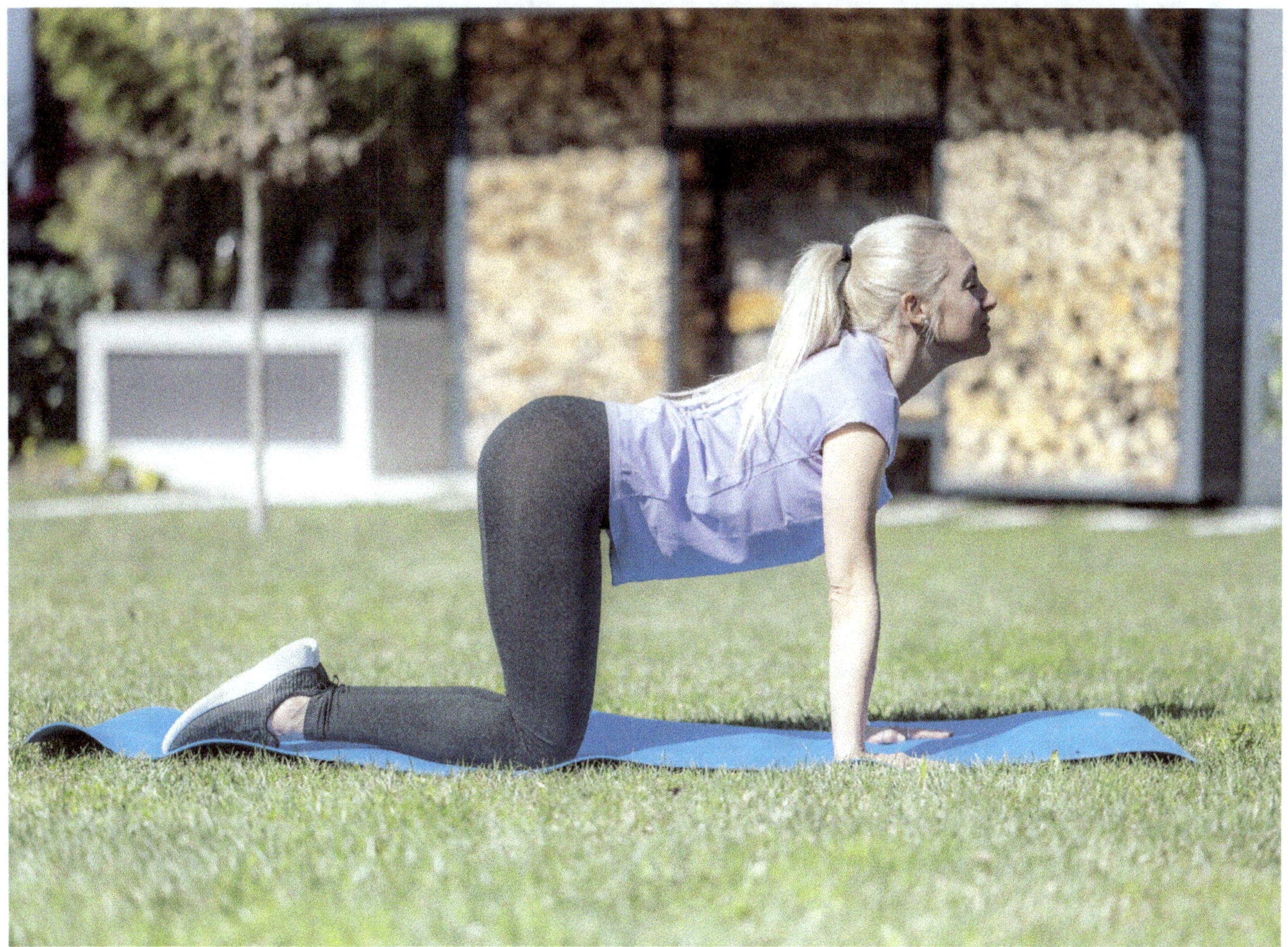

INSTRUCTIONS

- Start by positioning yourself on all fours in a tabletop stance, ensuring that your wrists are directly aligned under your shoulders and your knees are beneath your hips.
- As you inhale, gently arch your back into the cow pose, and as you exhale, smoothly round your back into the cat pose.
- Continue this sequence for 10 repetitions.

SAFETY TIPS

- Avoid overstretching or forcing movements.

- Perform a brief warm-up before starting to ensure muscles are ready for movement.

- If you have wrist or knee issues, use props or modify the position to suit your comfort.

PIRIFORMIS STRETCH

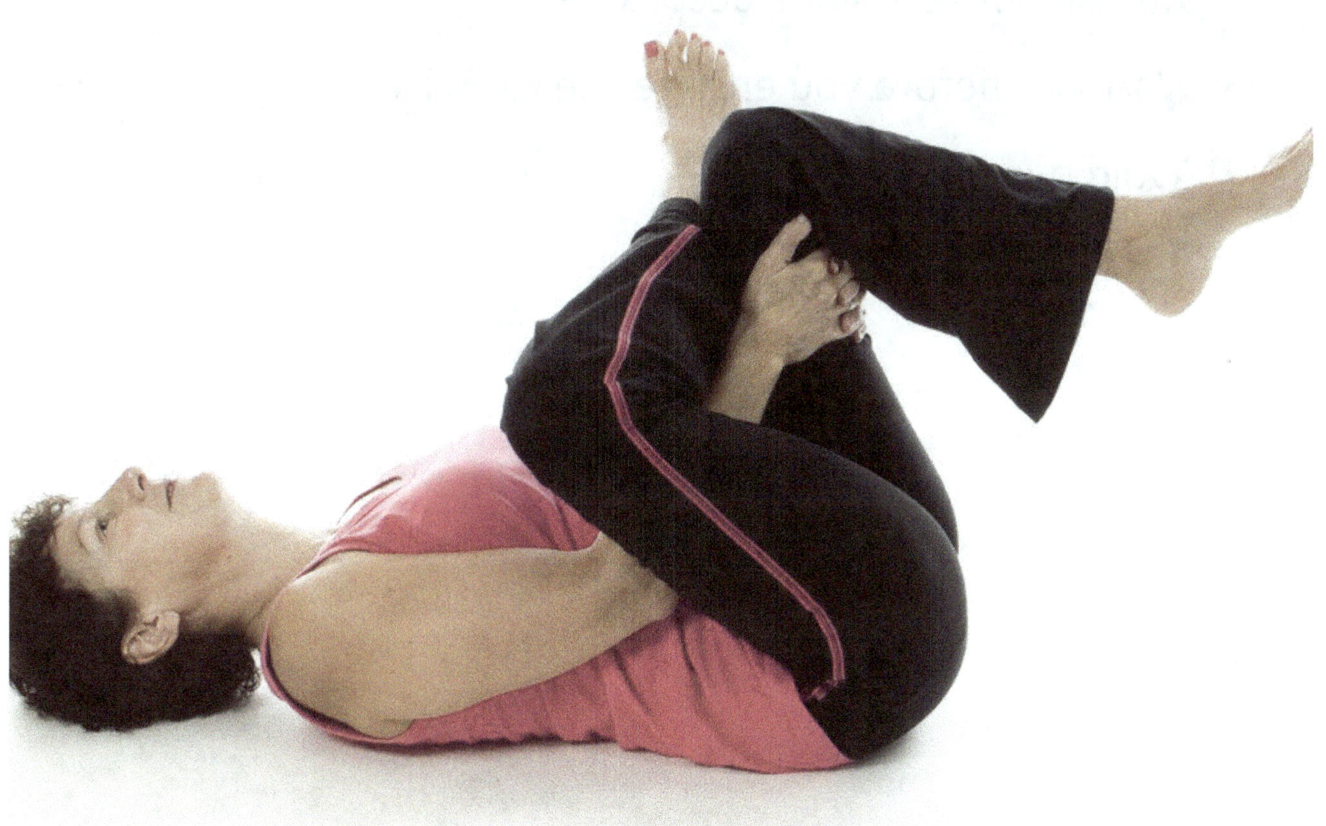

INSTRUCTIONS

- Rest the ankle of your upper leg over the knee of the other leg.

- Grasp the thigh and pull that knee toward your chest. You will feel a stretch along the buttocks and possibly along the outside of your hip on the other side.

- Hold this for 30 seconds. Repeat three times.

SAFETY TIPS

- Pay attention to any discomfort or pain and adjust the intensity or technique accordingly.

- Warm up before you engage the exercise

- Avoid overstretching

SIDE BEND STRETCH

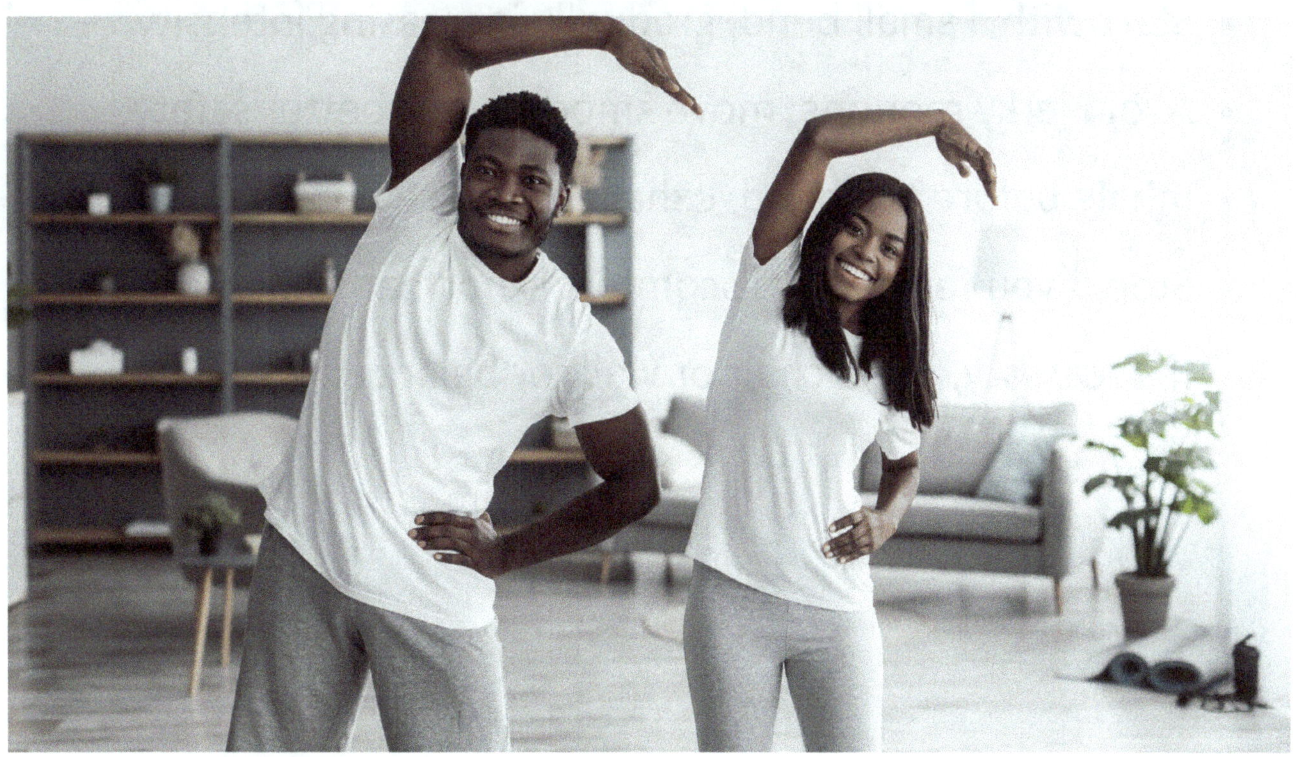

INSTRUCTIONS

- Stand with feet shoulder-width apart, knees slightly bent.

- Keep a straight spine, shoulders relaxed.

- Place hands on hips or clasp them together overhead. Inhale and gently lean to one side without twisting.

- Feel the stretch on the opposite side; hold for 15-30 seconds.

- Exhale, return to the upright position.

- Switch sides, perform 2-3 sets on each side.

SAFETY TIPS

- Start with a small bend, gradually increasing intensity.

- Avoid jerky motions; move smoothly for better safety.

- Inhale before the bend, exhale as you return.

- Stop if you feel pain; discomfort is normal, pain is not.

- If necessary, use a chair or wall for balance.

TRUNK ROTATION STRETCH

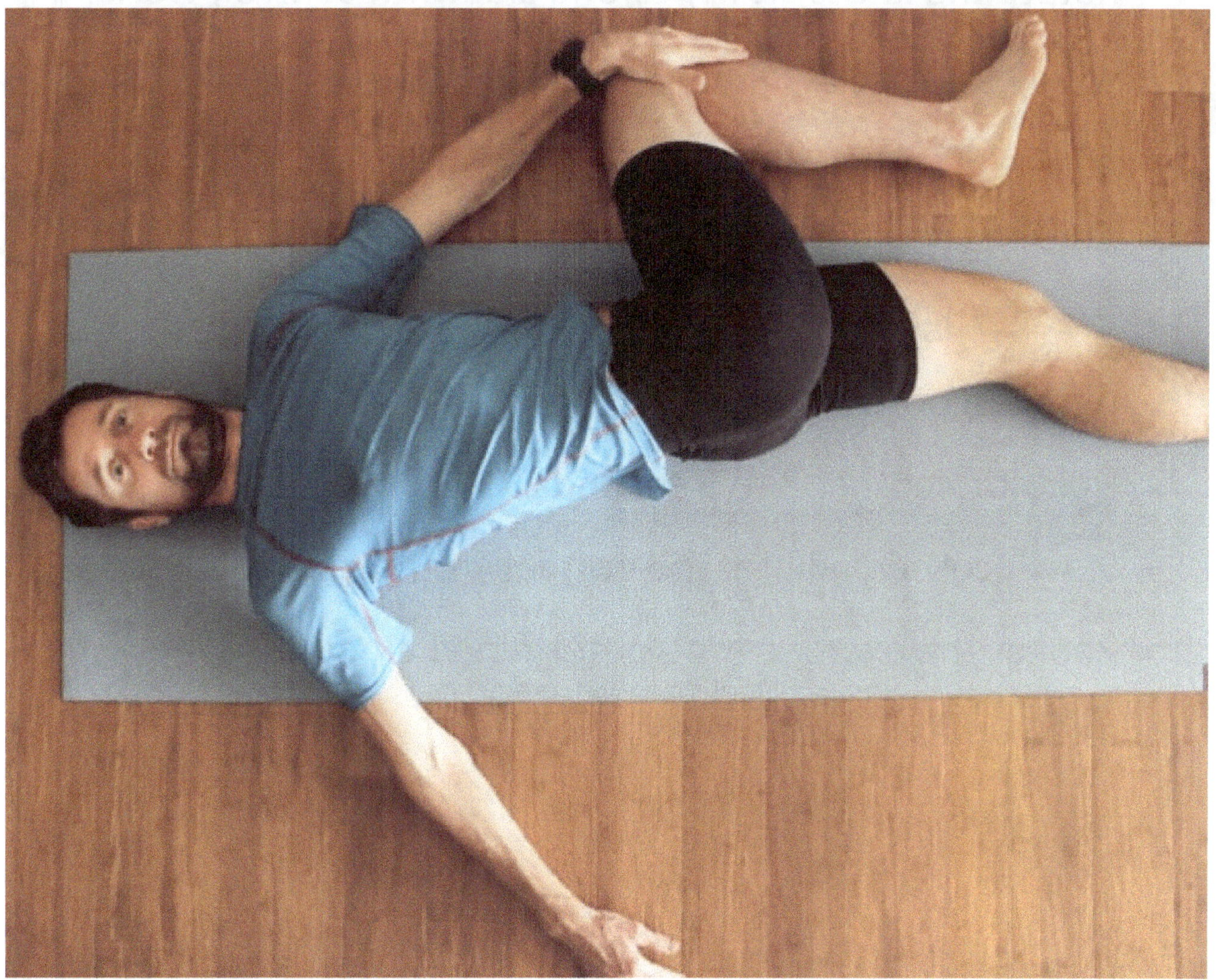

INSTRUCTIONS

- Start in a supine position (lying on back) on an exercise mat.

- Keep your knees bent and feet flat on the floor.

- Maintain your shoulders and upper body firmly against the floor.

- Outstretch your arms and press them into the floor to help with balance during the movement.

- Engage/tighten the abdominal muscles.

- Rotate the knees slowly to one side with control, working within your range of motion. Your feet will shift but remain on the floor.

- Hold the position for 3 to 5 seconds.

- Engage/tighten the abdominal muscles to move your legs to the opposite side.

- Hold for another 3 to 5 seconds.

- Stay focused and breathe normally through the exercise.

- Repeat the exercise for a determined amount of reps, such as 10 times on each side.

SAFETY TIPS

- Start with a gentle warm-up.

- Maintain proper posture throughout.

- Perform the exercise on a flat surface.

- Listen to your body.

BRIDGE POSE

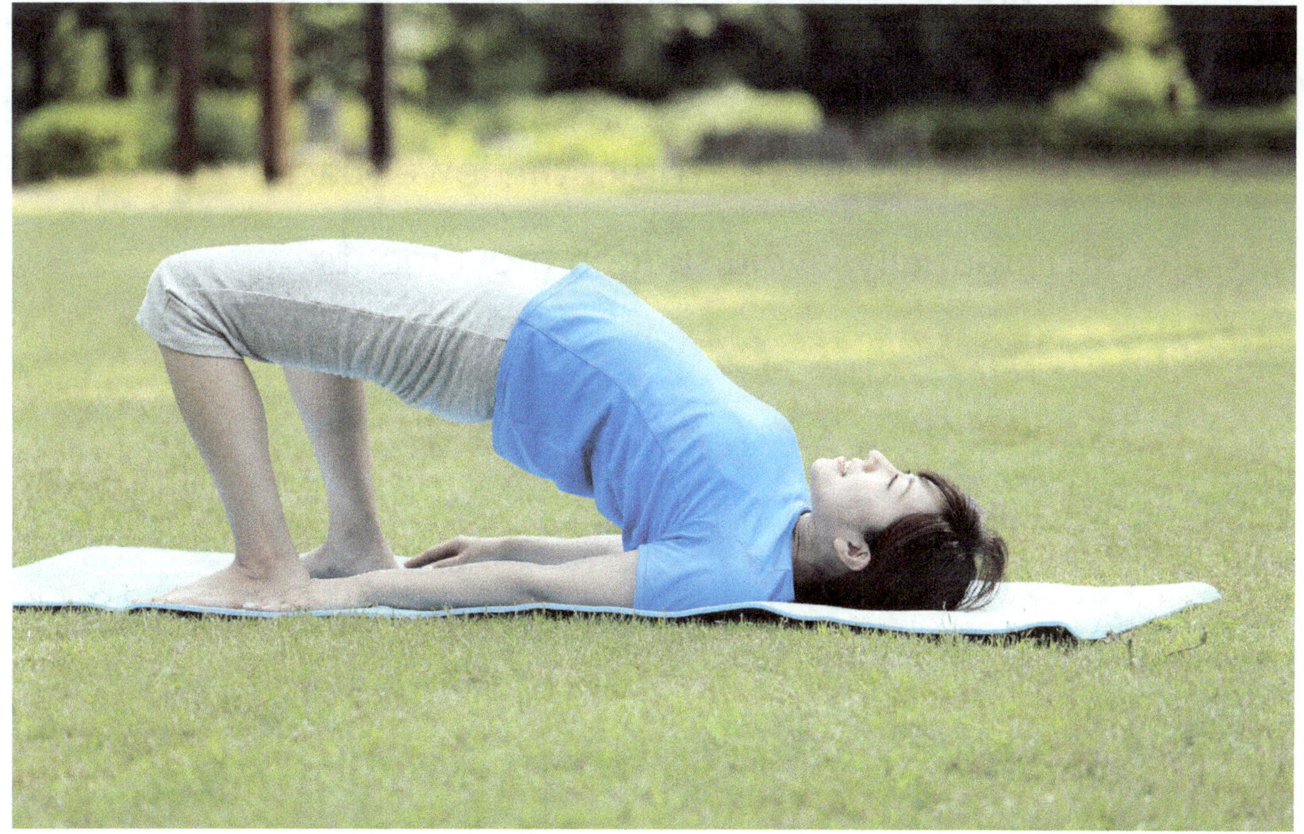

INSTRUCTIONS

- Begin by lying on your back with your knees bent and feet positioned hip-width apart.

- Push through your feet to raise your hips upward.

- Interlace your hands beneath your lower back and roll your shoulders back.

- Ensure your neck remains loose and your gaze is directed towards the ceiling.

SAFETY TIPS

- Avoid overextending your neck—keep it in a neutral position.

- Engage core muscles to protect the lower back.

- Lift hips gradually, avoid sudden movements.

STANDING FORWARD BEND

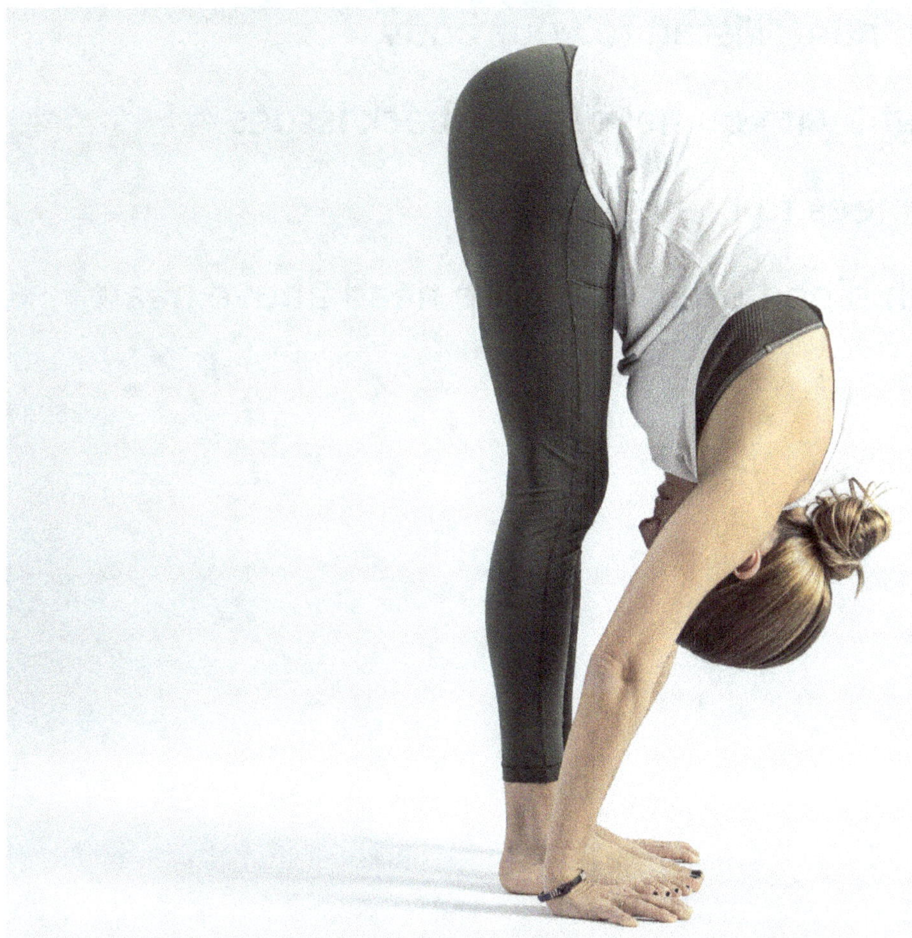

INSTRUCTIONS

- Stand with feet hip-width apart.

- Inhale, lift arms overhead.

- Exhale, hinge at hips, and fold forward.

- Keep spine straight, reaching hands towards the floor.

- Hold for 30 seconds to 1 minute, breathing deeply.

- Inhale, rise slowly.

SAFETY TIPS

- Don't push too hard, Listen to your body,

- Bend knees slightly if you have lower back issues.

- Avoid locking knees to prevent strain.

- If you have high blood pressure, keep head above heart level.

STANDING QUAD STRETCH

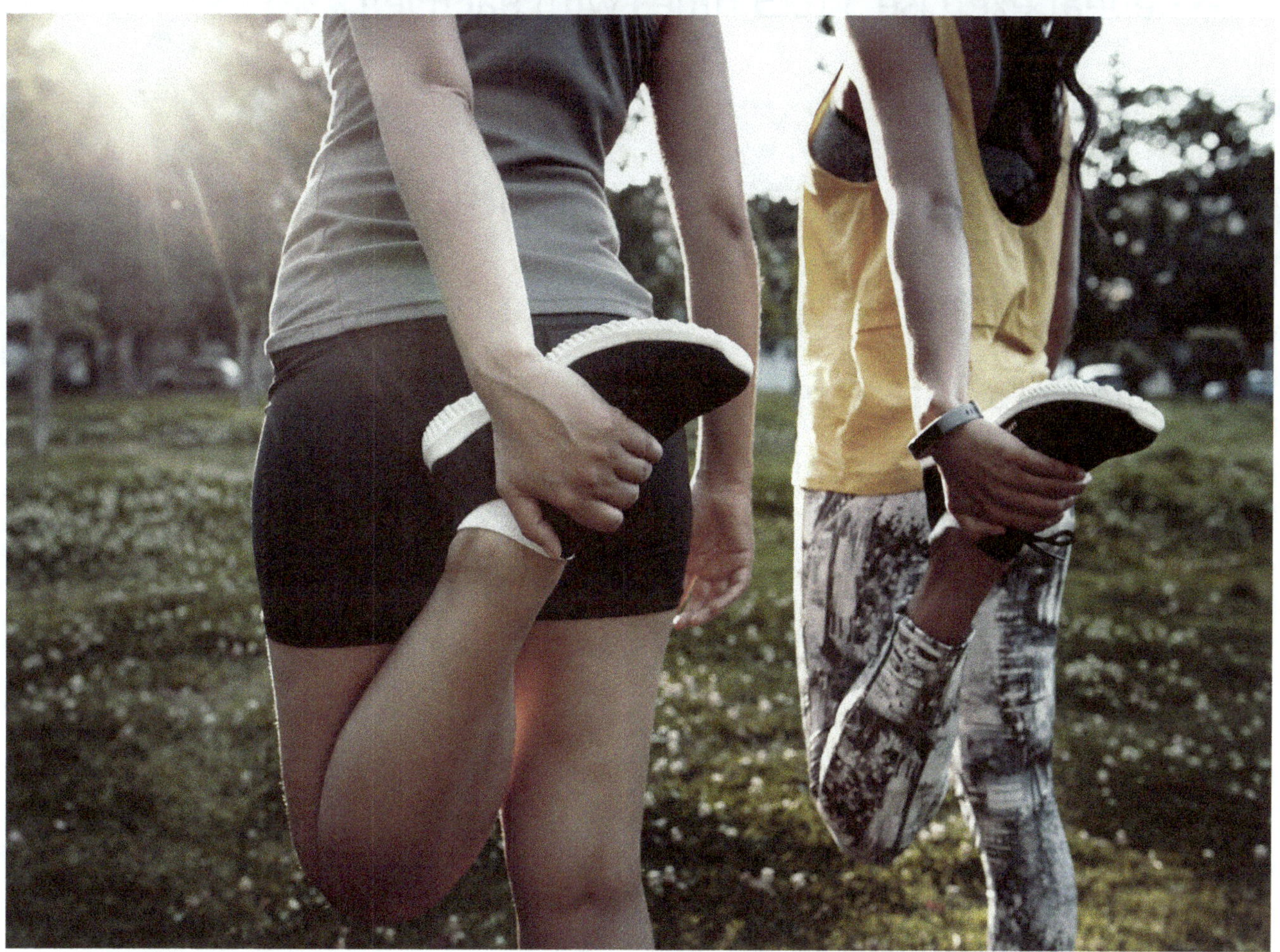

INSTRUCTIONS

- While standing, hold onto a countertop or chair back to assist in balance.

- Bend your knee by grasping your ankle with one hand, moving your foot toward your buttocks.

- Gently pull on your ankle to bend your knee as far as possible.

- Maintain position for 30 seconds.

- Return to standing position.

- Repeat exercise 3 to 5 times with each leg.

SAFETY TIPS

- Maintain balance by engaging your core.

- Hold onto a stable surface if needed.

- Avoid excessive pulling to prevent strain.

- Perform the stretch on both legs for balance.

- Listen to your body

SUPINE SPINAL TWIST

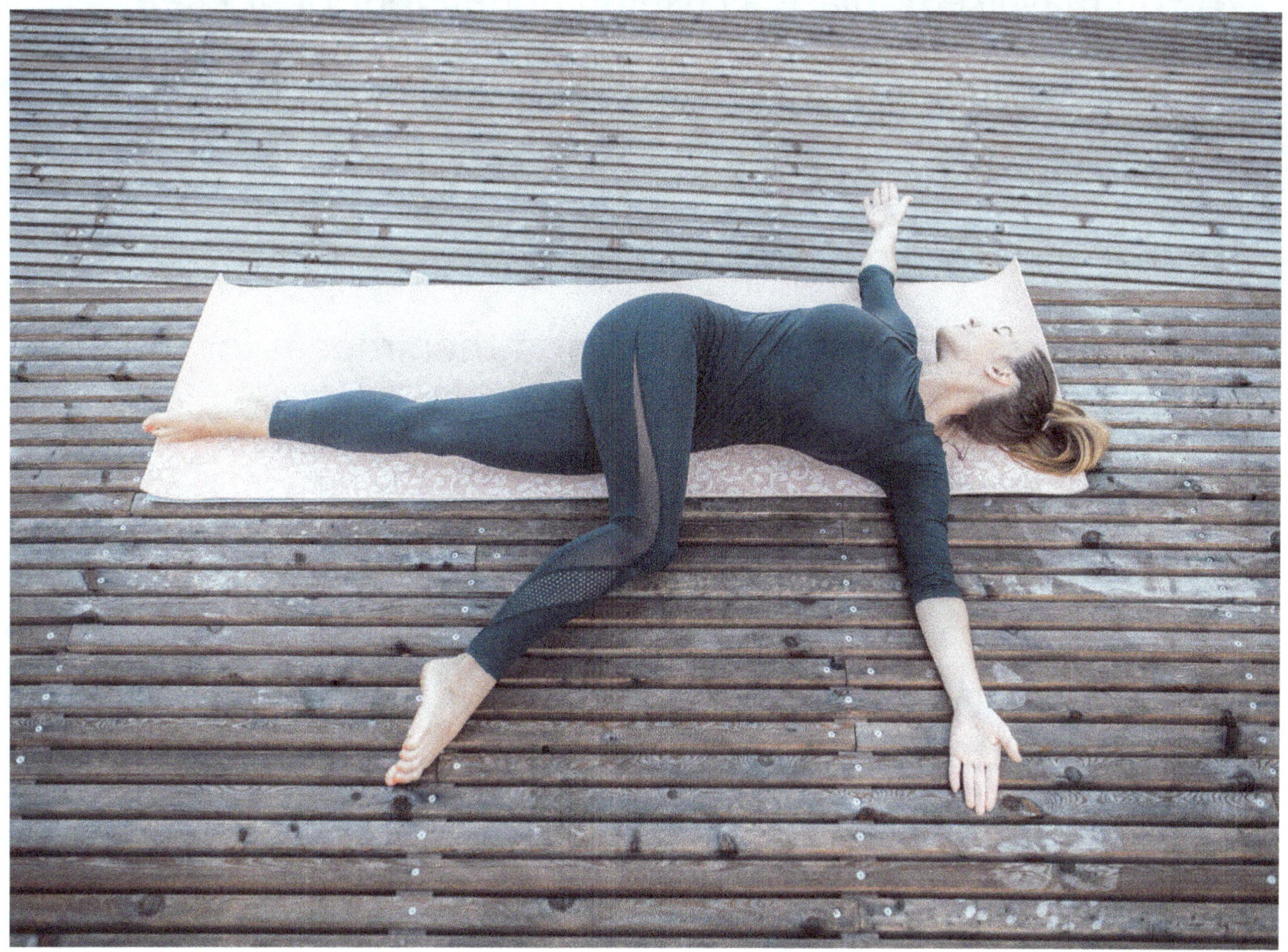

INSTRUCTIONS

- Lie on your back with your legs outstretched and arms spreading out in line with your shoulders.

- Shift your hips to the right of the mat.

- Bend your right knee and place the foot comfortably on the left thigh or behind the left knee

- Roll onto your left hip so the right hip is pointing towards the ceiling. If your right shoulder lifts also that's okay.

- Although ideally it stays on floor.

- You may like to place a cushion under your right knee and/or under your right shoulder.

- Turn your head to the right if comfortable.

- Breathe into all areas of your lungs and relax.

- Stay for as long 5 – 30 breaths and then repeat for the same amount on the other side.

SAFETY TIPS

- Start with lighter weights.

- Maintain proper form to avoid injuries.

- Consult a fitness professional if unsure.

- Listen to your body; don't push too hard.

- Warm up before attempting

COBRA POSE

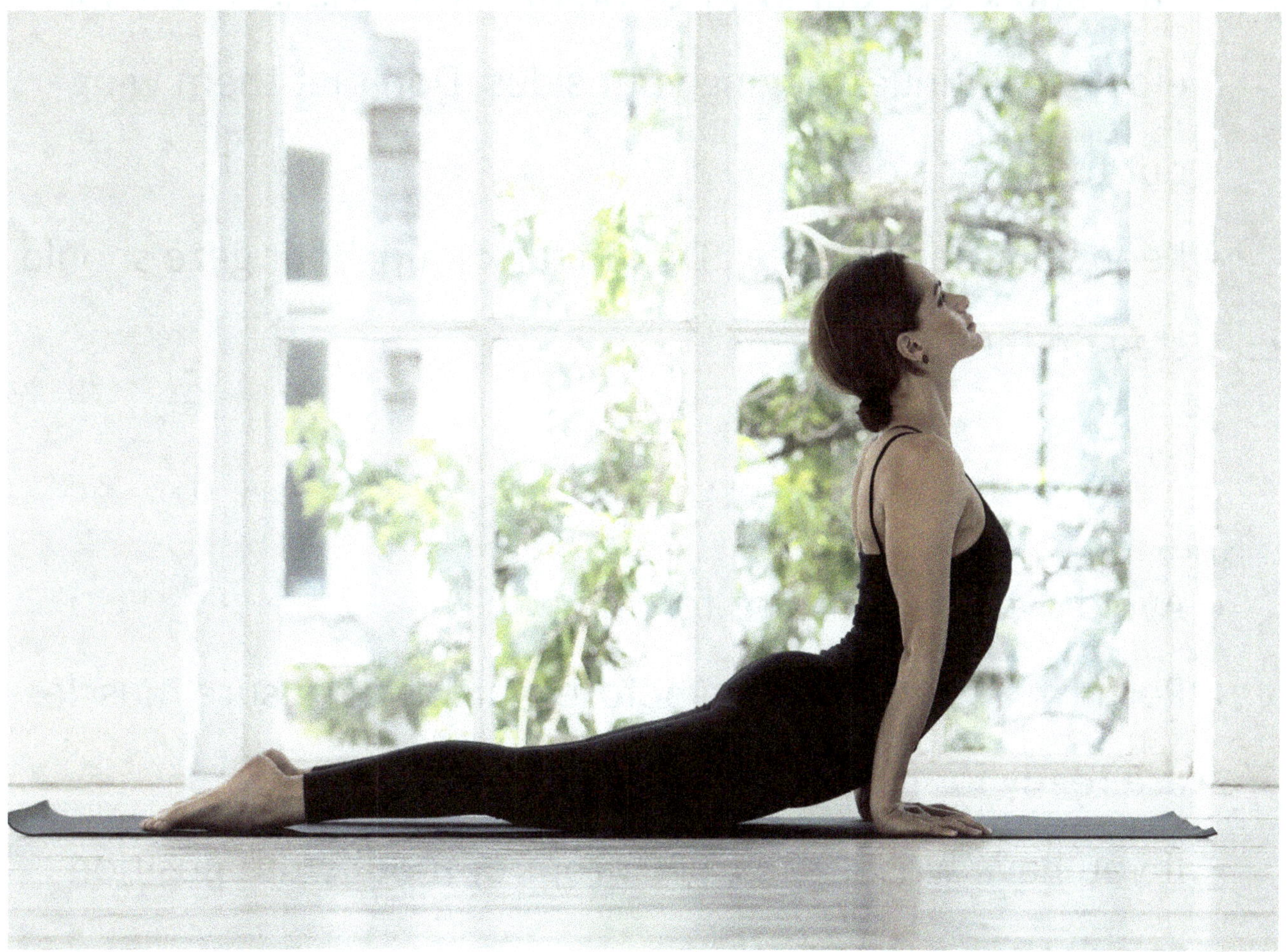

INSTRUCTIONS

- Place your palms flat on the ground directly under your shoulders. Bend your elbows straight back and hug them into your sides.

- Pause for a moment looking straight down at your mat with your neck in a neutral position. Anchor your pubic bone to the floor.

- Inhale to lift your chest off the floor. Roll your shoulders back and keep your low ribs on the floor. Make sure your elbows continue hugging your sides. Don't let them wing out to either side.

- Keep your neck neutral. Don't crank it up. Your gaze should stay on the floor.

SAFETY TIPS

- Avoid overstretching or forcing.

- Perform a brief warm-up before starting to ensure muscles are ready for movement.

- If you have wrist issues, use props or modify the position to suit your comfort.

STANDING LUNGE STRETCH

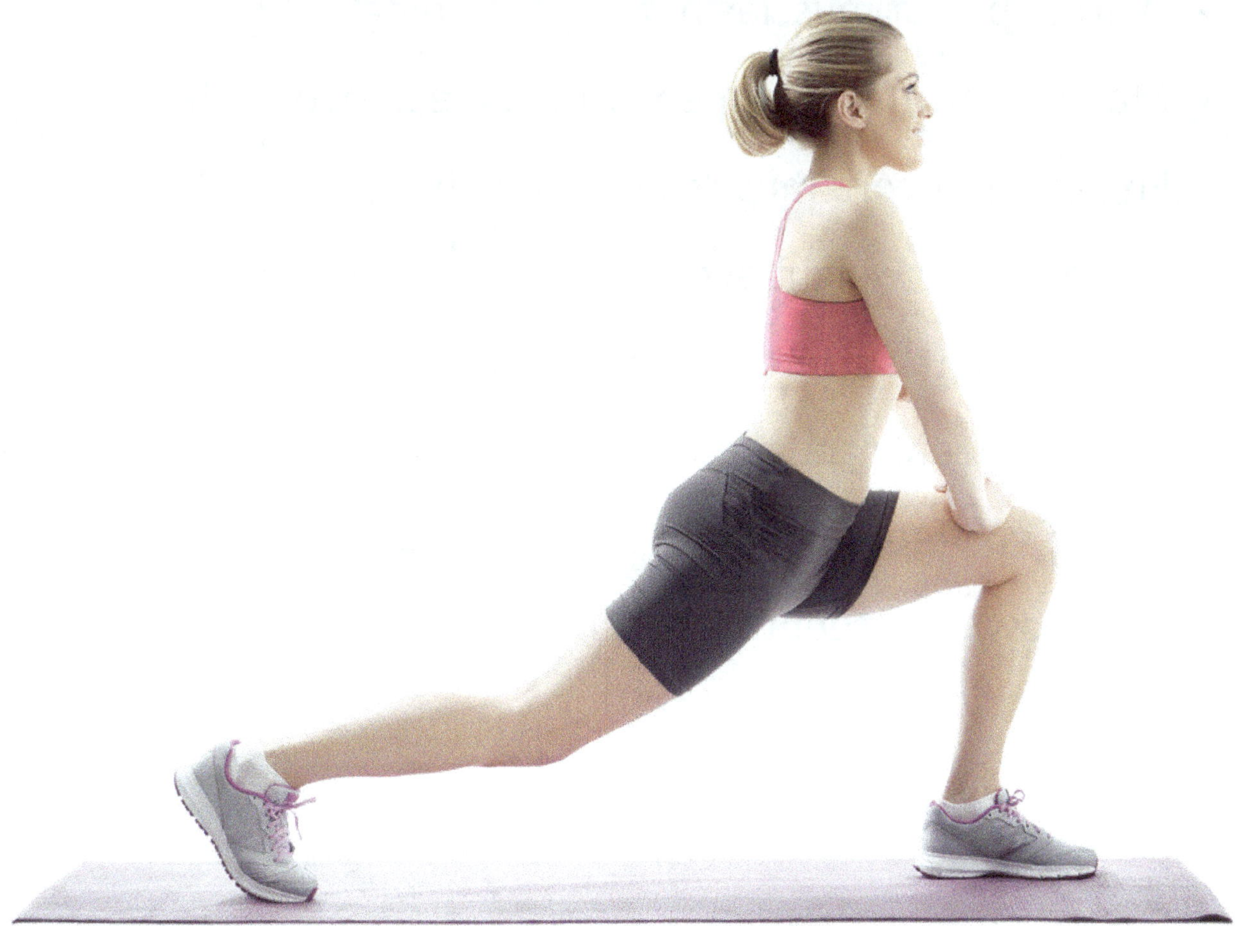

INSTRUCTIONS

- Stand up straight with your arms at your side.

- Place your hands on your hips or on your forward knee.

- Take a step forward with your right foot so you are standing in a split stance.

- Lower your right knee so it is at a 90-degree angle. Your left leg is extended straight back behind you.

- Hold the stretch for 20-30 seconds.

- Release and repeat on the other side.

42

SAFETY TIPS

- Warm up your muscles before stretching.

- Maintain proper alignment with knee above ankle.

- Engage your core muscles for stability.

- Balance your weight evenly between both feet.

- Lower into the stretch slowly and avoid bouncing.

- Breathe deeply and steadily throughout the stretch.

- Stop if you feel sharp pain and listen to your body.

- Cool down with gentle stretches afterward.

DOWNWARD FACING DOG

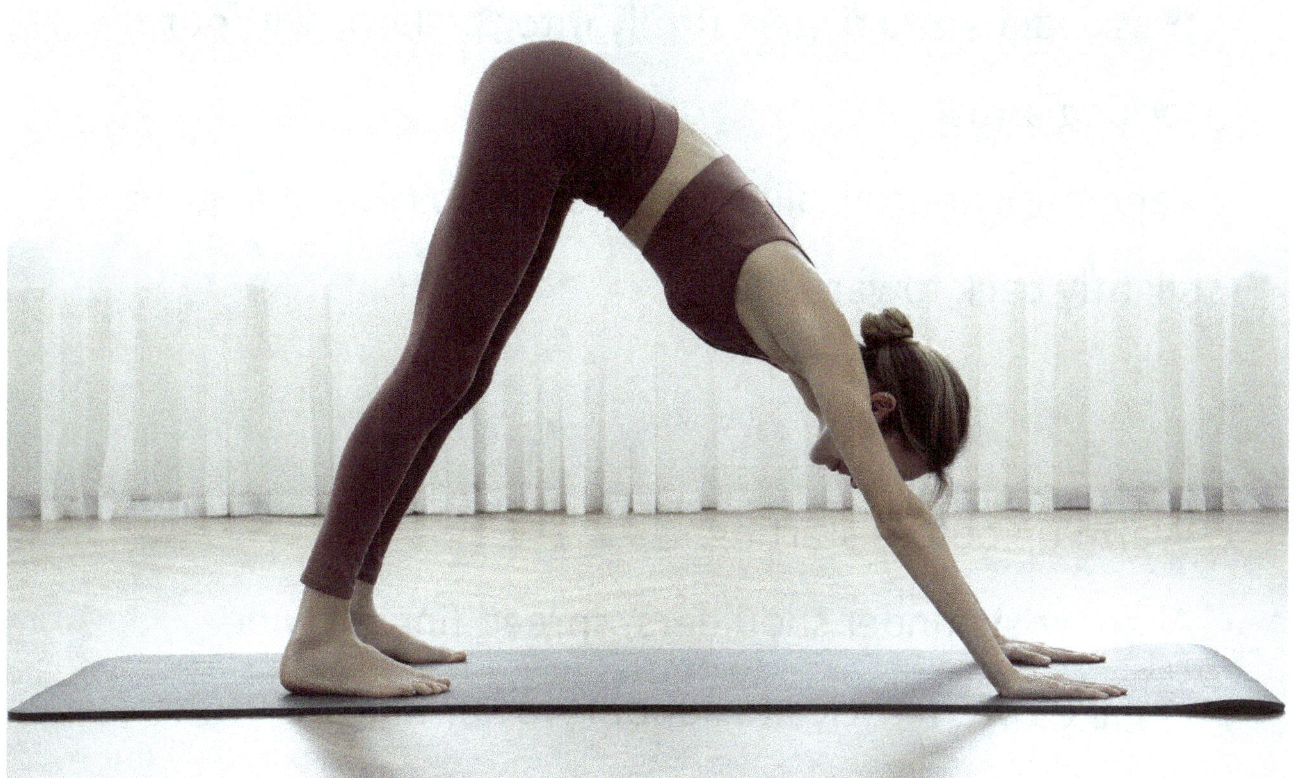

INSTRUCTIONS

- Start on hands and knees, with hands shoulder-width apart and fingers spread wide.

- Lift knees off the floor, sending hips upward while exhaling.

- Straighten legs gradually, without locking knees, and lower heels toward the ground.

- Tilt sitting bones upward and rotate inner thighs slightly inward and upward.
- Draw ribs gently in by engaging the belly.
- Press palms and fingers firmly into the floor without locking arms.
- Keep neck neutral, aligning ears with biceps, and gaze slightly back toward feet.

SAFETY TIPS

- Warm up before starting.
- Align wrists under shoulders, spread fingers wide.
- Engage core muscles to support lower back.
- Lengthen spine, lift hips toward ceiling.
- Modify with bent knees or props if needed.
- Listen to your body; avoid pain or discomfort.
- Focus on steady breathing.

THREAD THE NEEDLE STRETCH

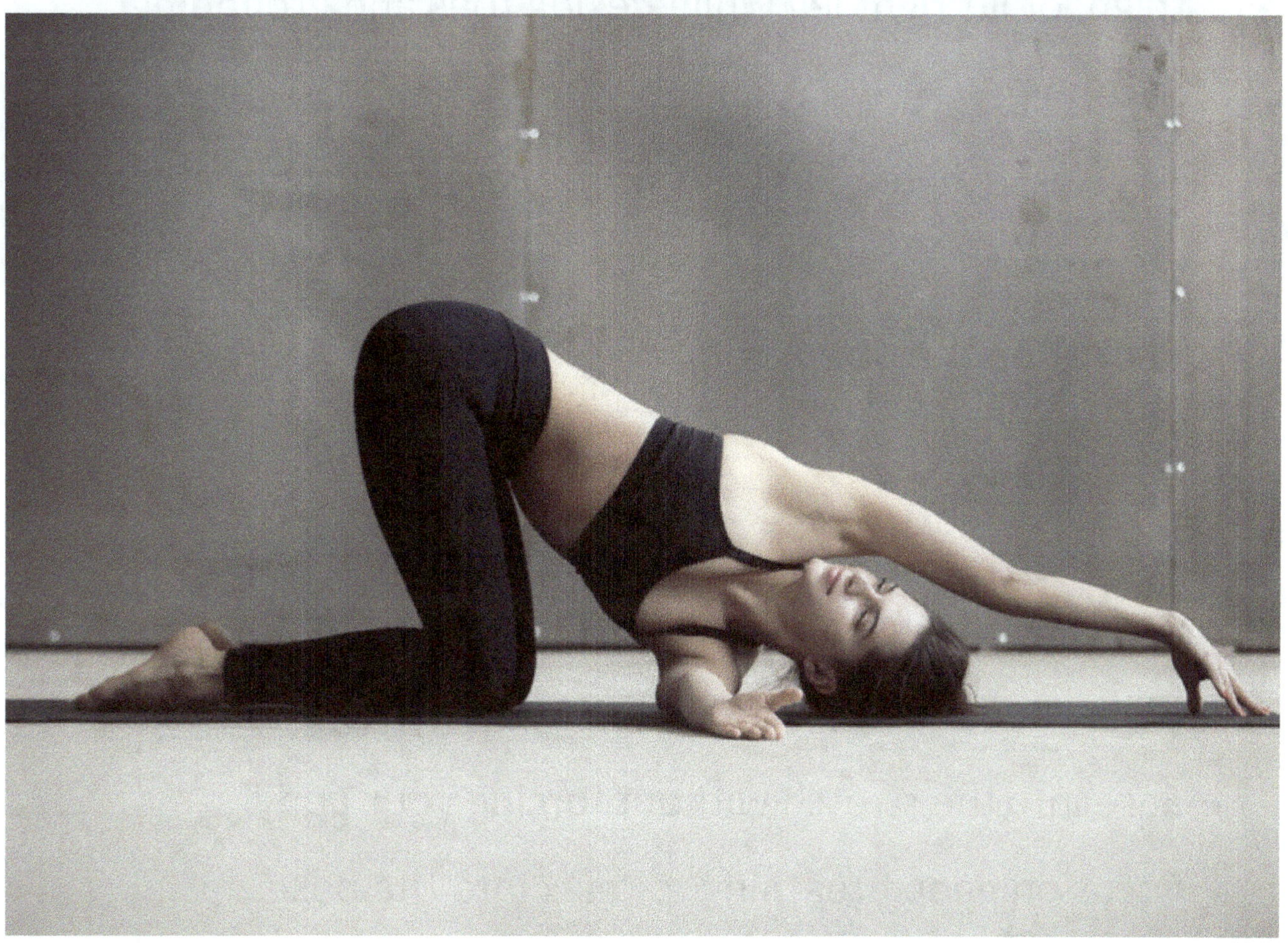

INSTRUCTIONS

- Start on all fours with hips directly above knees.

- Hands shoulder-width apart, spread fingers wide, engage core.

- Inhale, lift right arm up, gaze follows.

- Exhale, thread right arm under left, left arm extends forward, right cheek to ground, gaze left.

- Optionally, bring left arm to lower back, grab right inner thigh, or lift right leg while flexing toes and grounding outer hip.
- To release, extend both arms forward, return to tabletop position.
- Repeat on the other side.

SAFETY TIPS

- Always warm up your body before attempting the pose.
- Align your shoulders and wrists properly to avoid strain.
- Ease into the stretch without forcing your body.
- Focus on deep breathing to relax into the pose.
- Use props or modify the pose if you feel discomfort.
- Respect your body's limits and avoid overstretching.
- Practice regularly to improve flexibility and strength.

EAGLE POSE

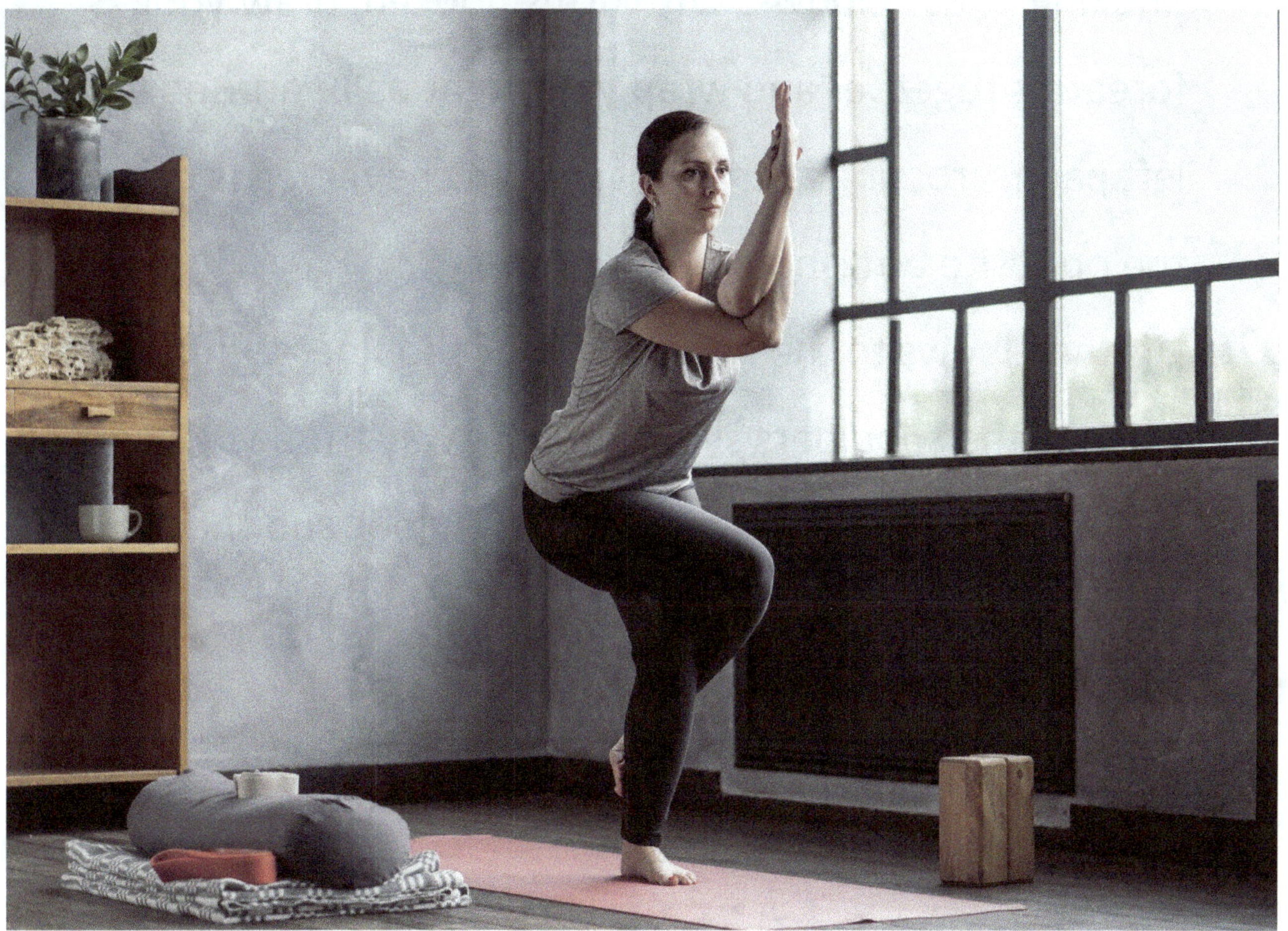

INSTRUCTIONS

- Transfer your weight into your left foot.

- Lift your right foot up off the floor.

- Cross your right thigh over your left thigh as high up the thigh as possible.

- Hook your right foot around your left calf.

- Bring both arms out in front of you and parallel to the floor.

- Bend your arms and cross the left arm over the right, hooking at the elbows. With arms hooked, draw your forearms together and wrap your right palm around your left palm, crossing at the wrists. (Whichever leg is on top, the opposite arm should be on top.)
- Lift the elbows to the height of your shoulders while keeping the shoulders sliding down away from your ears.
- Keep your spine perpendicular to the floor and the crown of the head rising.
- Hold for 5 to 10 breaths.
- Repeat on the other side.

SAFETY TIPS

- Always warm up your body before attempting the pose.
- Align your shoulders and wrists properly to avoid strain.
- Ease into the stretch without forcing your body.
- Focus on deep breathing to relax into the pose.
- Use props or modify the pose if you feel discomfort.
- Respect your body's limits and avoid overstretching.
- Practice regularly to improve flexibility and strength.

SPHINX POSE

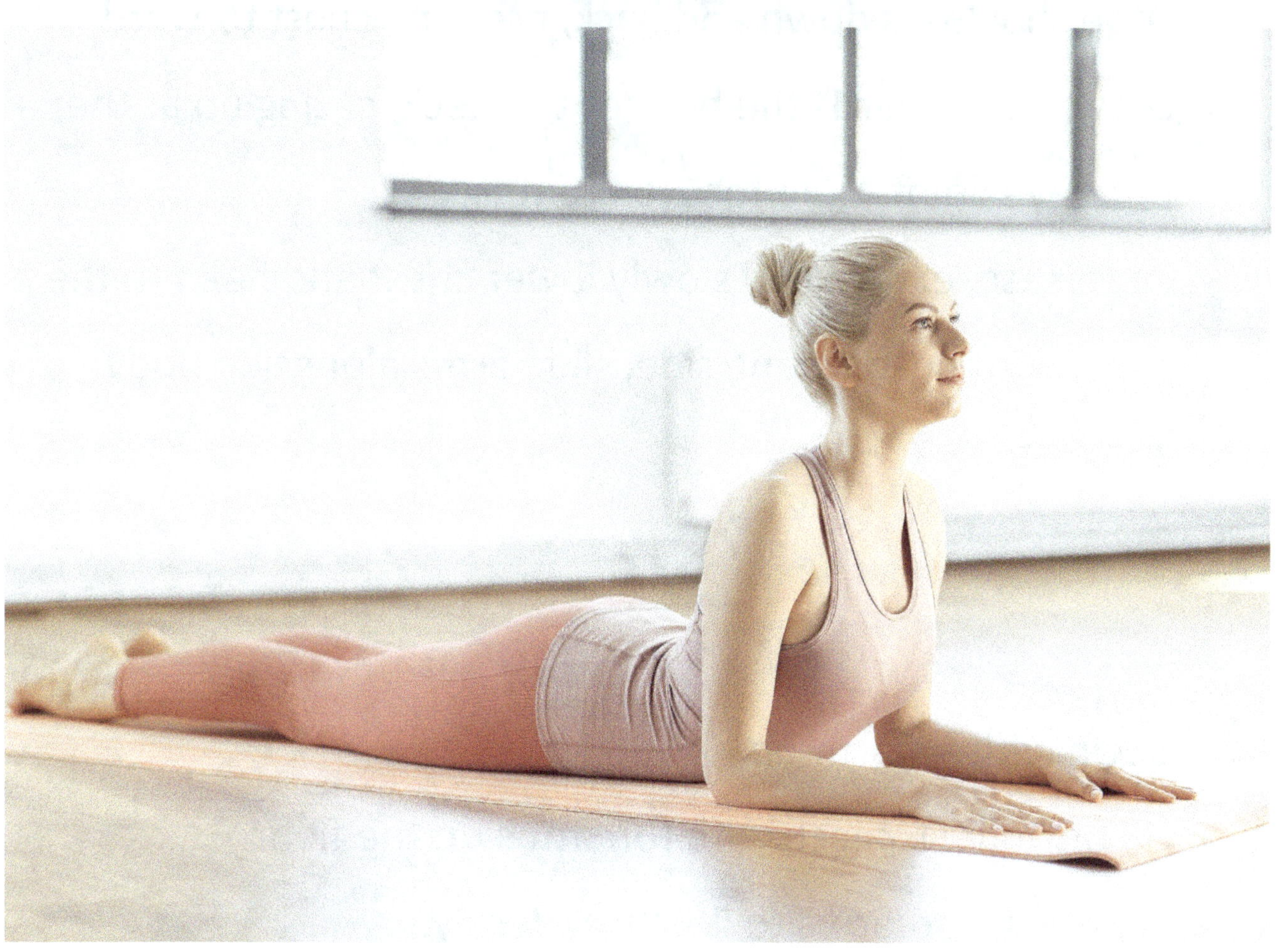

INSTRUCTIONS

- Start by lying on your belly, with forearms flat on the floor, elbows under shoulders, chin on the floor, and legs together.

- Inhale and lift head and chest off the floor, keeping neck aligned with the spine.

- Engage leg muscles, buttocks, and mula bandha (pelvic floor), while pressing pubic bone into the floor.

- Keep elbows close to sides, using arms to lift chest higher. Drop shoulders down and back, pressing chest forward.
- Draw chin towards the back of the neck, gazing up at the third eye point. Hold for 2-6 breaths.
- To release, exhale and slowly lower chest and head to the floor. Turn head to one side, slide arms alongside body, and rest.

SAFETY TIPS

- Begin with a warm-up.
- Lie on your stomach with forearms on the floor.
- Press into forearms to lift chest gently.
- Engage core and relax shoulders.
- Hold, breathe deeply, and listen to your body.
- Modify if needed to avoid discomfort.
- Slowly release back down after holding.

DOWNWARD FACING DOG

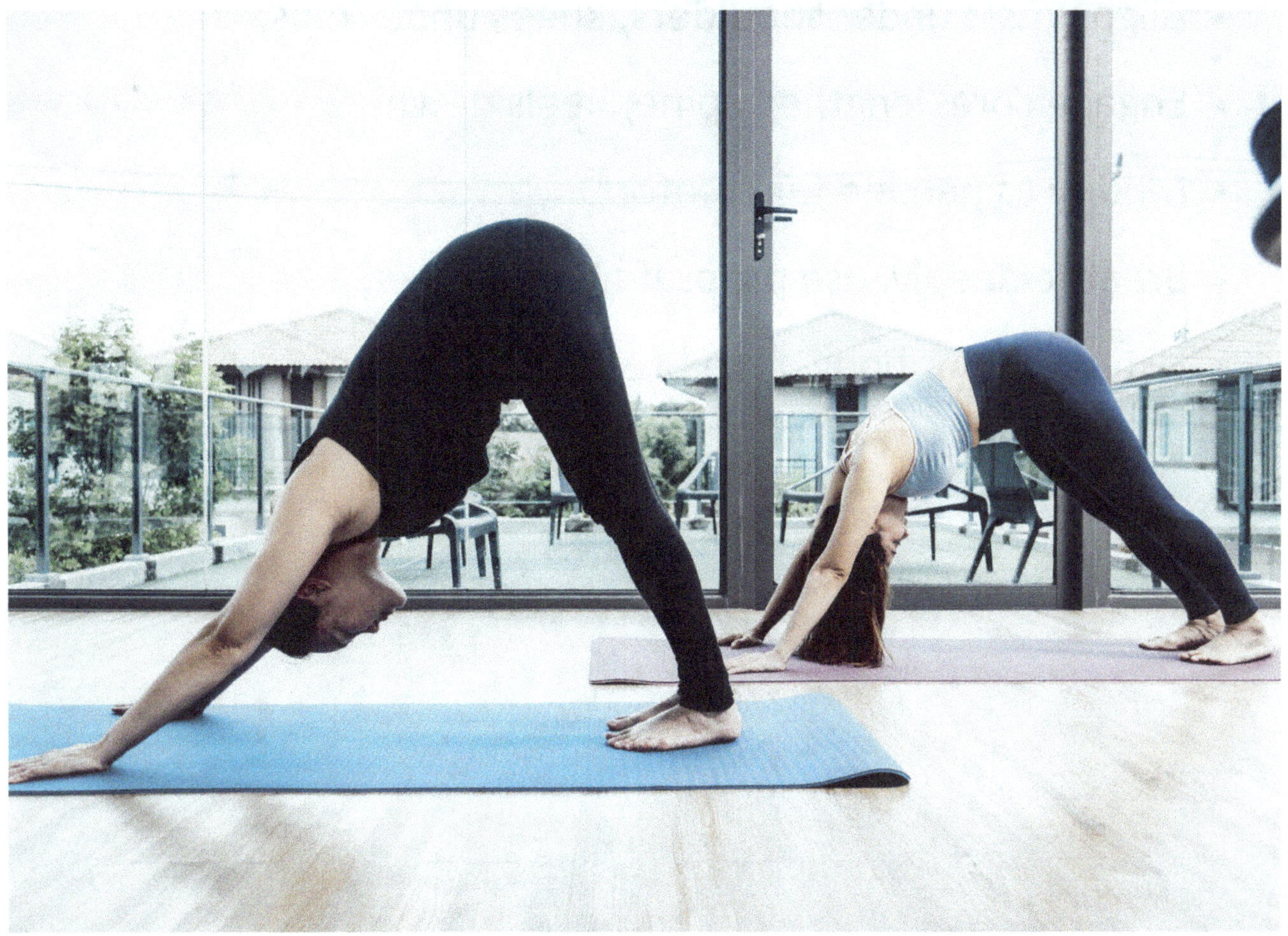

INSTRUCTIONS

- Start on your hands and knees.

- Lift your hips towards the ceiling, straightening your arms and legs, forming an inverted V shape.

- Press your hands into the mat, lengthen your spine, and engage your core. Keep your heels reaching towards the ground.

SAFETY TIPS

- Align wrists under shoulders, knees under hips.

- Engage core, lengthen spine, heels down.

- Modify as needed for comfort.

- Breathe deeply, use props if helpful.

- Listen to your body, take breaks if necessary.

UPWARD FACING DOG

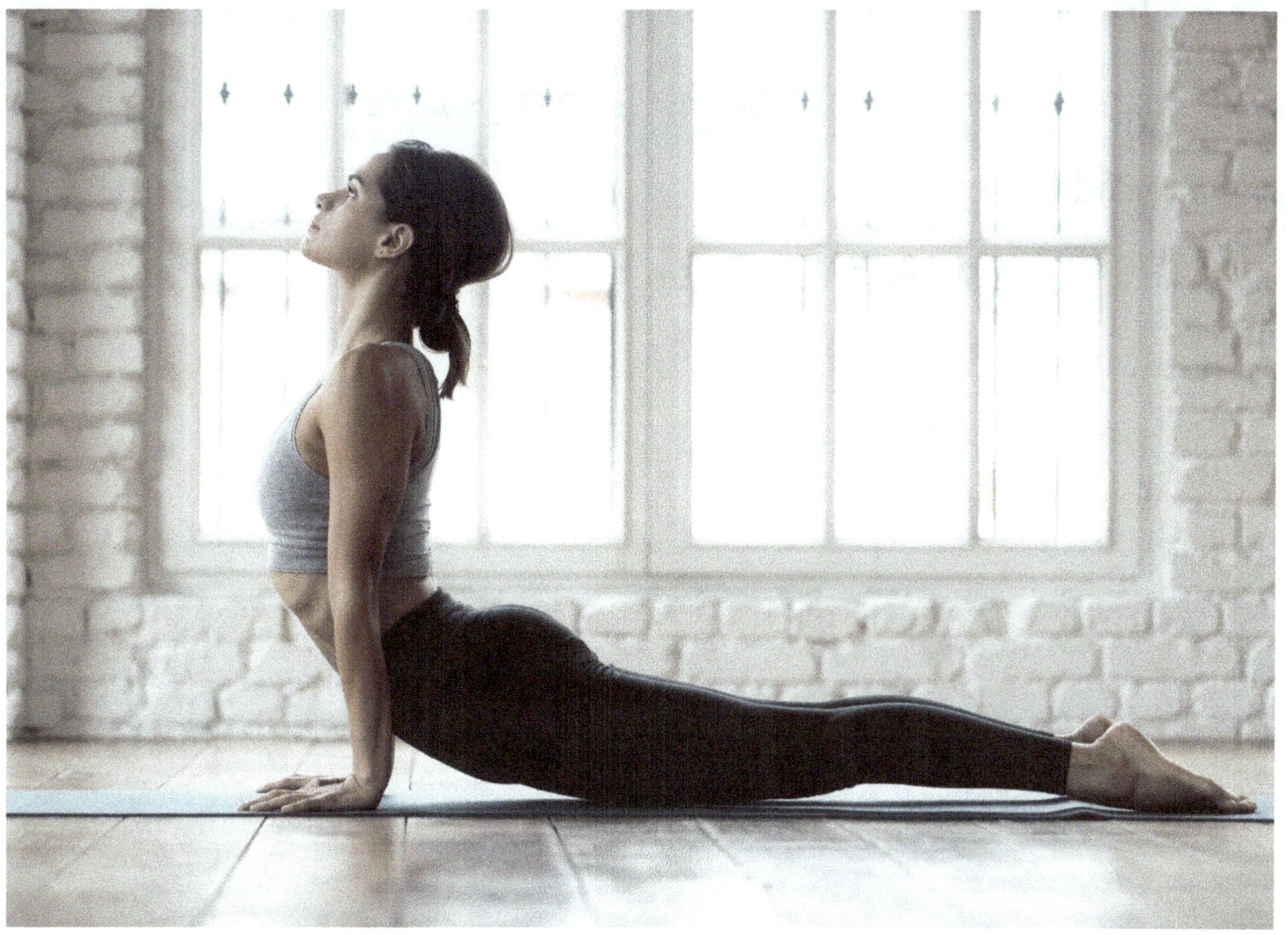

INSTRUCTIONS

- Lie face down on the mat with your hands positioned by your lower ribs.

- Press into your palms and lift your chest off the mat, straightening your arms.

- Keep your shoulders down and away from your ears, and engage your core to protect your lower back

SAFETY TIPS

- Warm up.

- Align hands under shoulders, engage core.

- Avoid lower back strain.

- Distribute weight evenly on hands.

- Modify for wrist comfort.

- Listen to your body, no pain.

- Breathe steadily.

PIGEON POSE

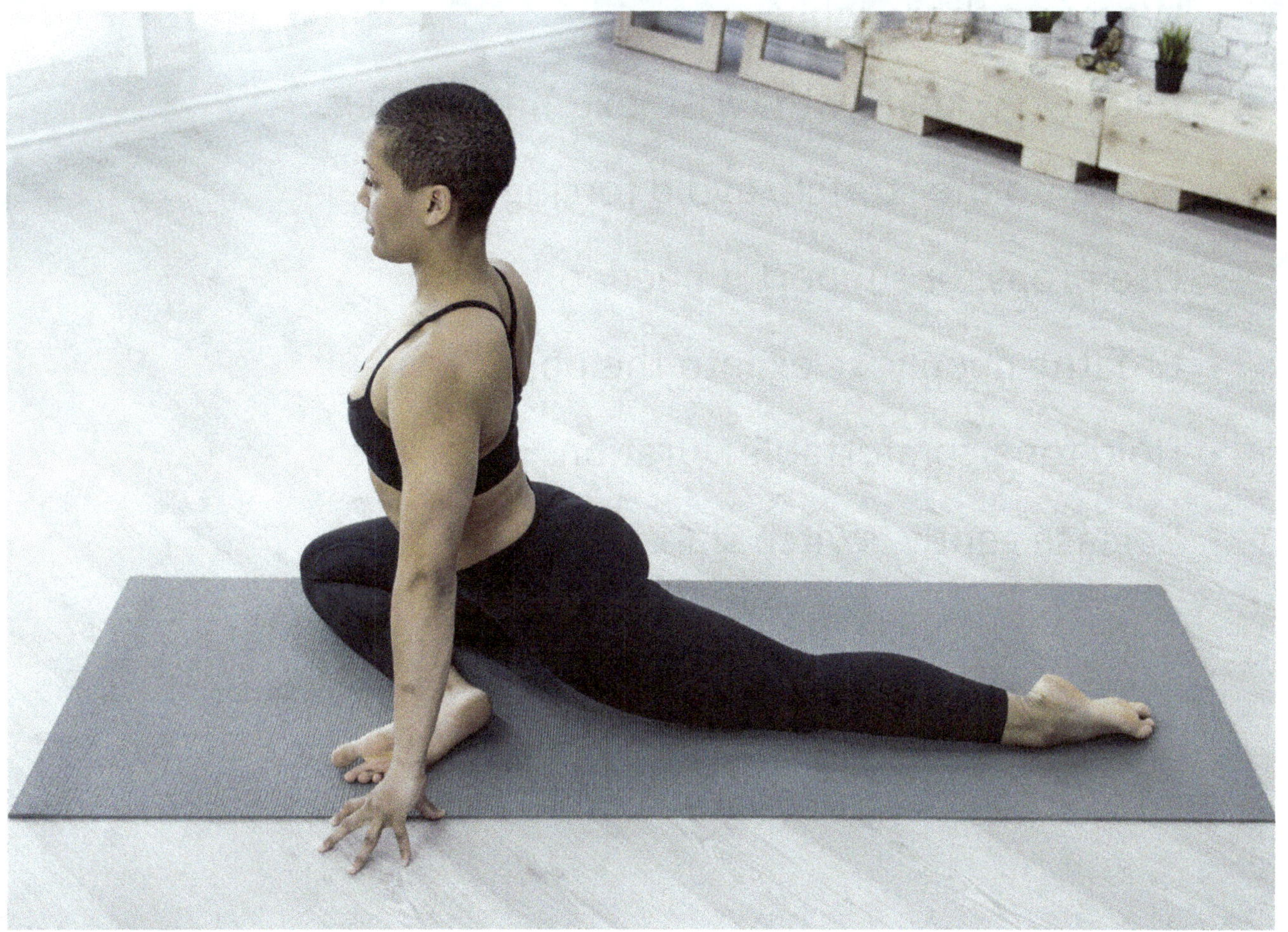

INSTRUCTIONS

- Start in a tabletop position.

- Bring one knee forward towards the same-side wrist, and extend the other leg behind you.

- Square your hips as much as possible, then walk your hands forward and lower your chest towards the ground.

SAFETY TIPS

- Warm up thoroughly.

- Align front knee with wrist, extend back leg.

- Ease into the stretch, avoid forcing.

- Use props for support if needed.

- Breathe deeply, relax into the pose.

- Hold for a comfortable duration.

- Release gently, switch sides.

EXTENDED TRIANGLE POSE

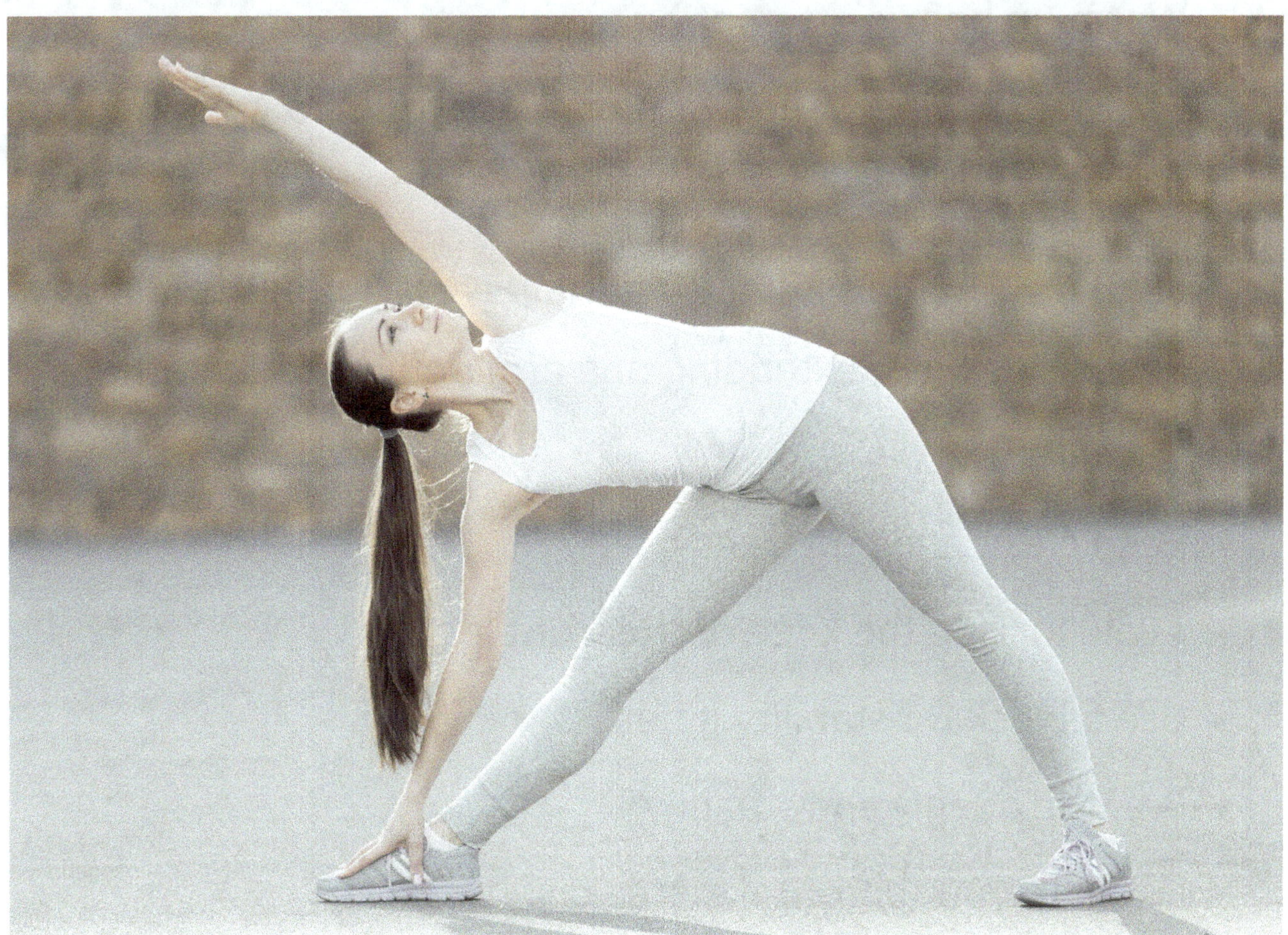

INSTRUCTIONS

- Begin in a standing position with feet wide apart.

- Turn one foot out and extend your arms parallel to the floor.

- Reach towards the extended foot with one hand while extending the other arm towards the ceiling, keeping your torso lengthened.

SAFETY TIPS

- Warm up before attempting.
- Maintain a wide stance with one foot forward and one foot back.
- Keep front foot pointed forward, back foot slightly angled.
- Reach sideways, extending one arm down and the other up.
- Keep chest and hips open.
- Avoid locking the knee of the front leg.
- Use a block for stability if necessary.
- Breathe deeply and steadily.
- Listen to your body, take breaks if necessary.

WARRIOR II POSE

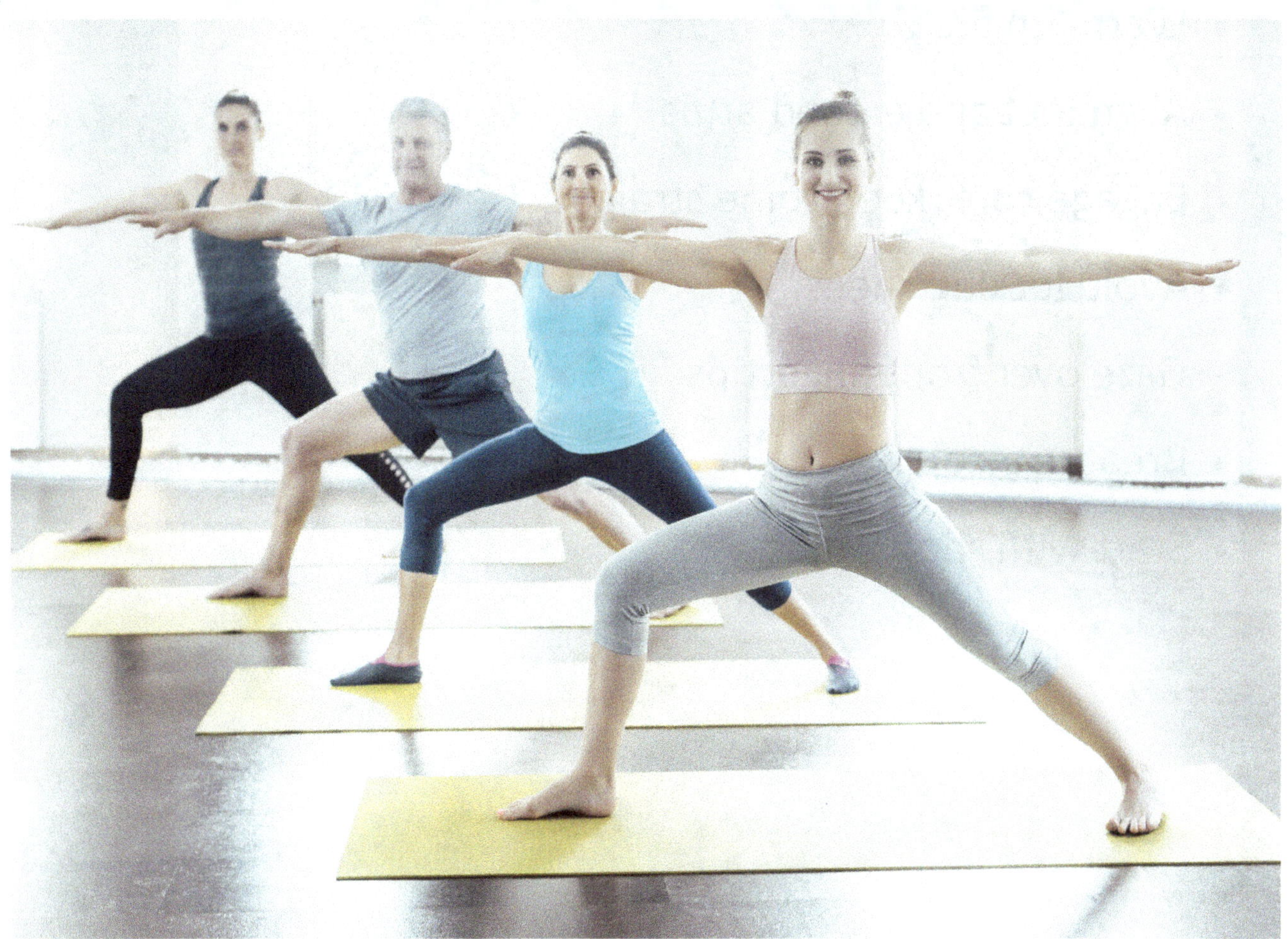

INSTRUCTIONS

- Start in a standing position with feet wide apart.

- Turn one foot out and bend the knee, aligning it with the ankle.

- Extend your arms parallel to the floor, gaze over the front fingertips, and sink into the front thigh while keeping the back leg straight.

SAFETY TIPS

- Warm up first.

- Align feet and extend arms.

- Engage core, keep spine straight.

- Avoid locking knees.

- Gaze over front fingertips.

- Breathe steadily.

- Start with short holds.

LOCUST POSE

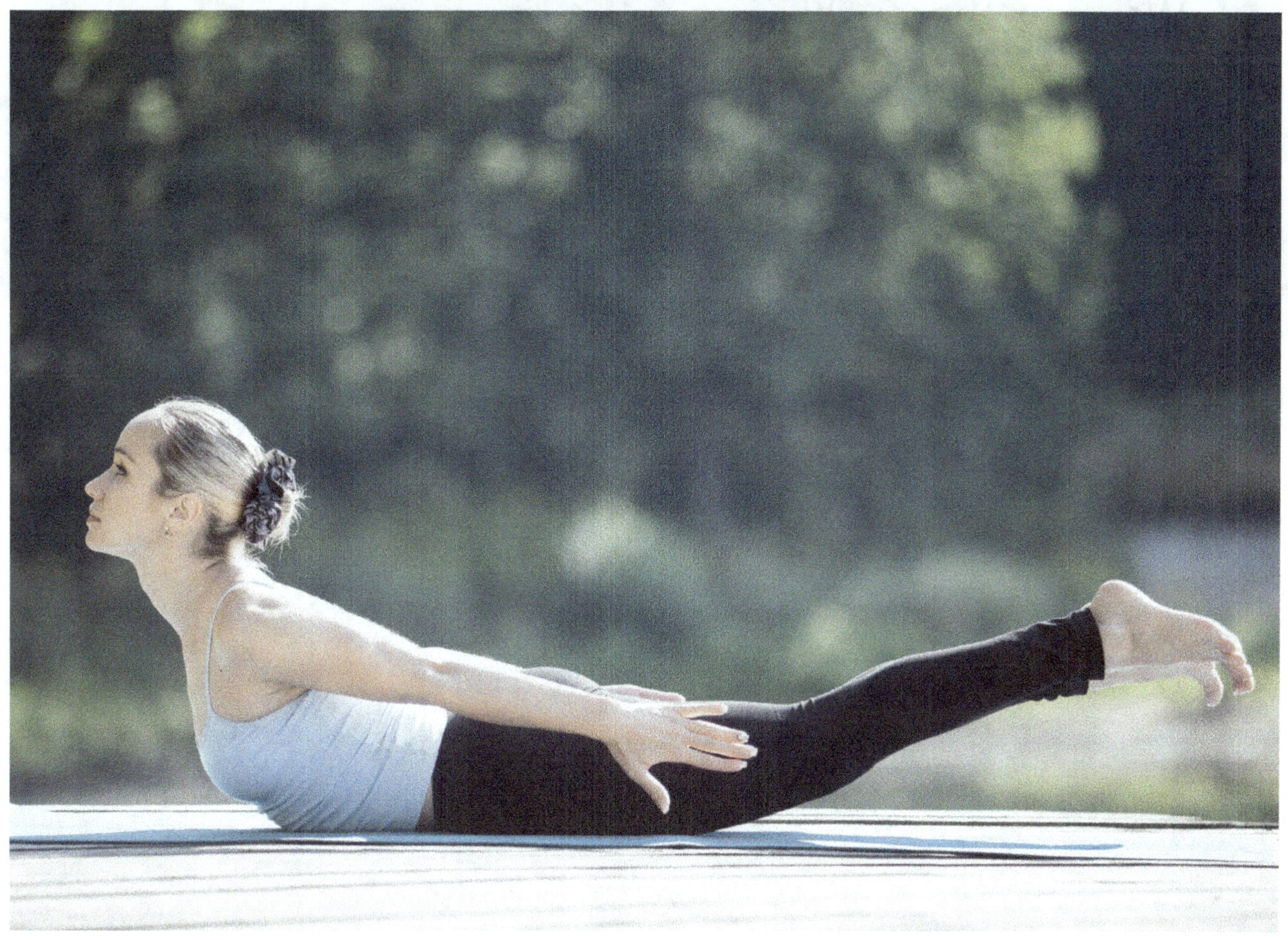

INSTRUCTIONS

- Lie on your stomach with your arms by your sides.

- Inhale, lift your chest, arms, and legs off the mat, engaging your back muscles.

- Keep your gaze forward and the back of your neck long.

SAFETY TIPS

- Warm up thoroughly.

- Align arms along body, palms down.

- Engage core and lift legs and chest.

- Avoid straining neck; gaze down.

- Support lower back; don't compress.

- Breathe steadily throughout.

CORPSE POSE

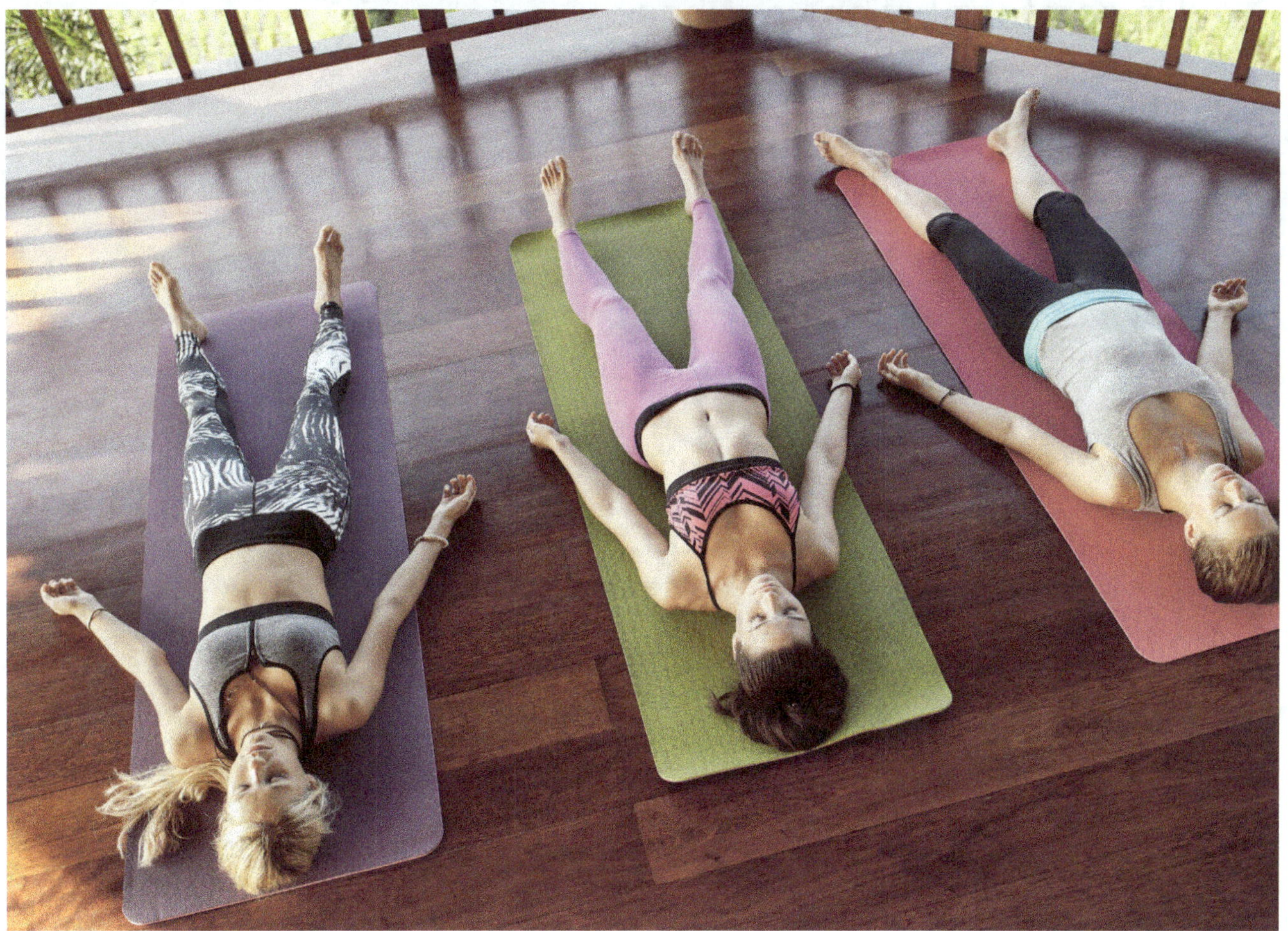

INSTRUCTIONS

- Lie flat on your back with your arms by your sides and palms facing up.

- Close your eyes and relax your entire body, allowing yourself to surrender to the mat and focus on your breath.

SAFETY TIPS

- Lie comfortably on your back.

- Relax your entire body.

- Breathe naturally.

- Stay present and mindful.

- Use props for support if needed.

- Stay warm with a blanket.

- Gradually increase duration.

- Exit slowly and mindfully.

HAPPY BABY POSE

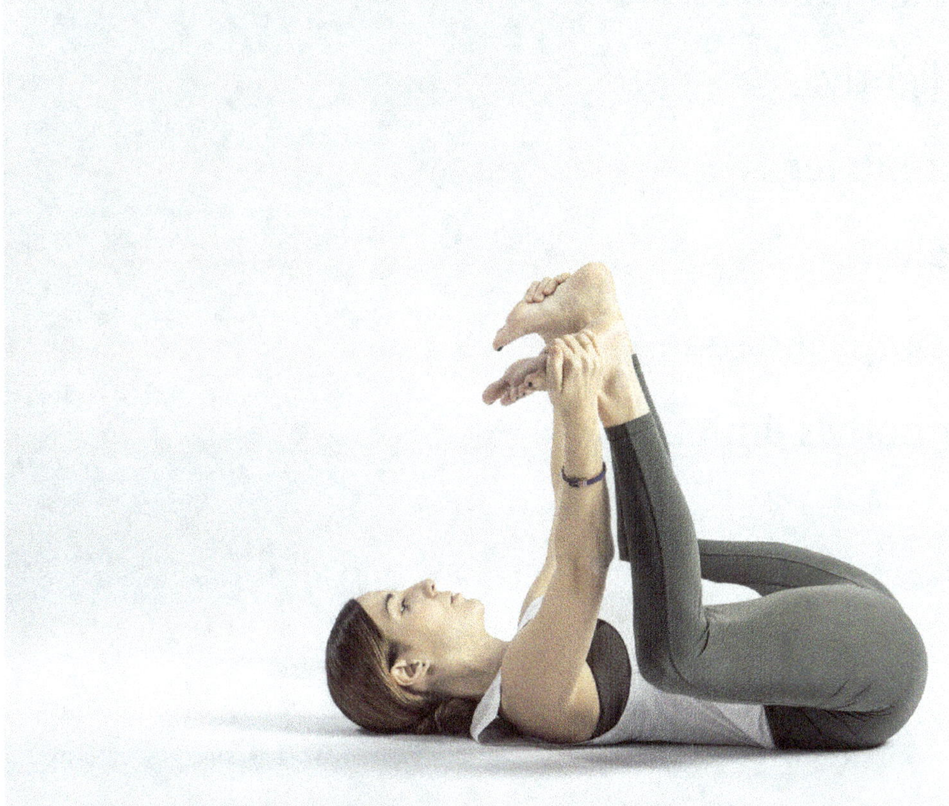

INSTRUCTIONS

- Lie on your back and draw your knees towards your chest.

- Grab the outer edges of your feet with your hands, and gently pull your knees towards your armpits.

- Keep your tailbone grounded as you lengthen through your spine.

SAFETY TIPS

- Gently stretch knees towards armpits.

- Relax neck and shoulders.

- Engage core lightly.

- Don't overextend legs.

- Breathe deeply.

- Modify with props if needed.

- Respect your body's limits.

SUPPORTED FISH POSE

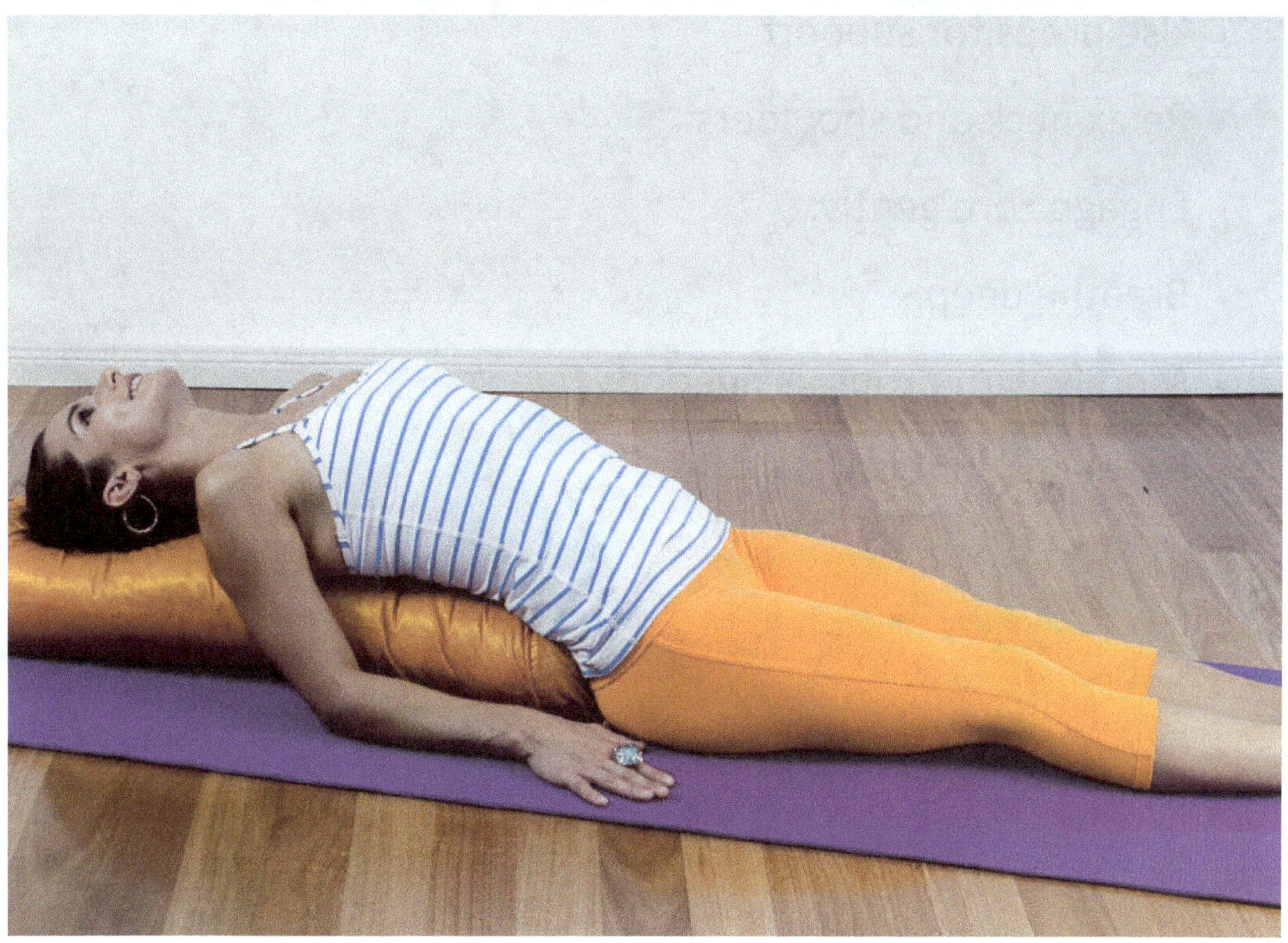

INSTRUCTIONS

- Place a yoga block or bolster horizontally on the mat.

- Sit in front of the prop with your knees bent and feet flat on the mat.

- Slowly recline back onto the prop, allowing your chest to open and your head to rest comfortably.

SAFETY TIPS

- Use props for support.

- Relax neck and shoulders.

- Engage core gently.

- Breathe deeply.

- Modify with props as needed.

- Respect your body's limits.

GARLAND POSE

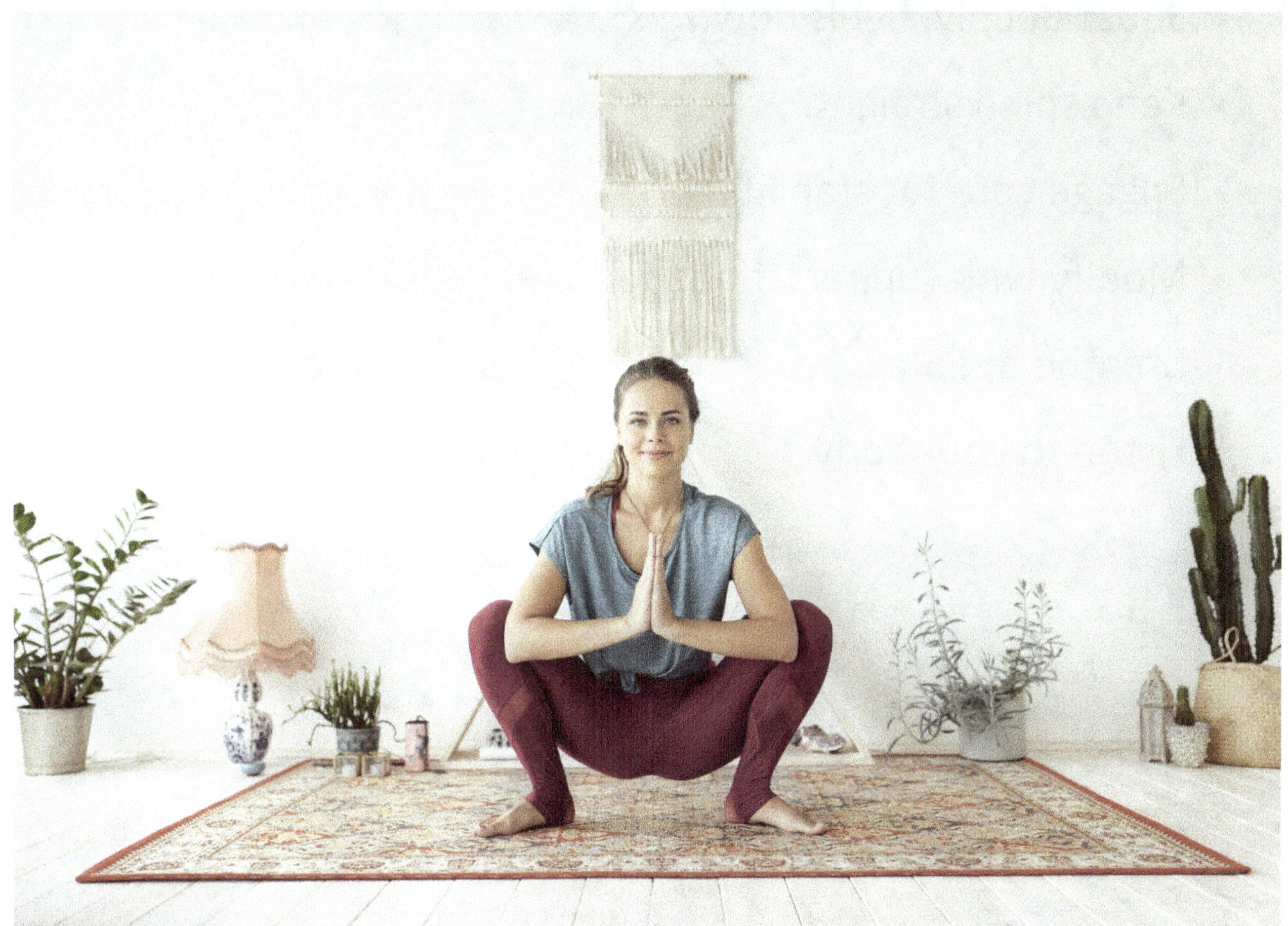

INSTRUCTIONS

- Start standing with your feet wider than hip-width apart.

- Squat down, bringing your hips towards your heels while keeping your heels grounded.

- Bring your palms together at your heart center and press your elbows against your inner thighs to help open your hips.

SAFETY TIPS

- Squat deeply, heels down.

- Keep spine straight.

- Engage core for stability.

- Modify with support if needed.

- Breathe deeply.

- Listen to your body

STANDING SIDE STRETCH

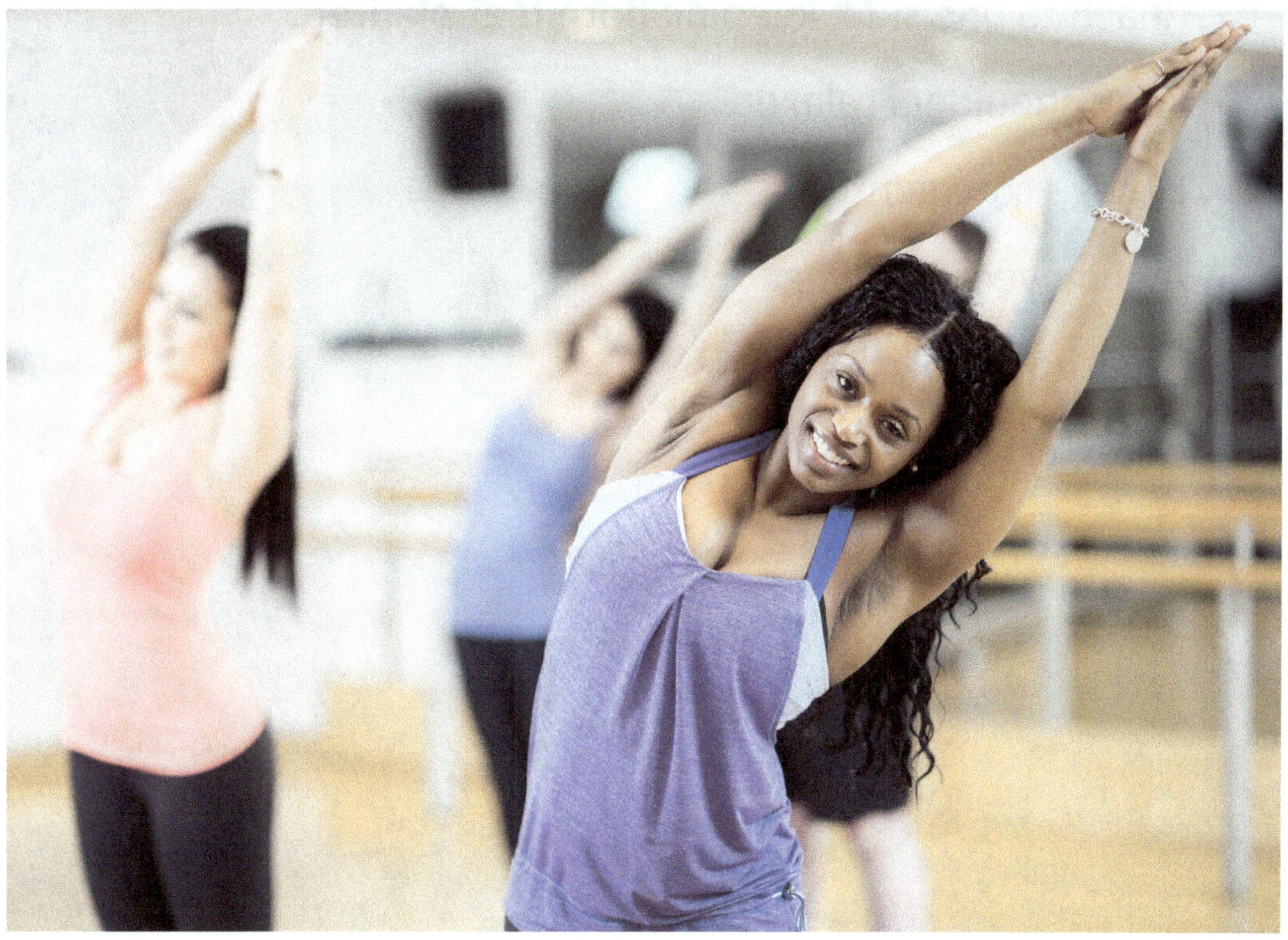

INSTRUCTIONS

- Stand with your feet hip-width apart and arms by your sides.

- Inhale, reach your arms overhead, and clasp your hands together.

- Lean to one side, elongating your torso and creating space between your ribs and hips.

SAFETY TIPS

- Reach to one side, keeping both feet planted.

- Keep shoulders relaxed.

- Engage core gently.

- Avoid overstretching.

- Breathe deeply.

- Listen to your body.

HALF LORD OF THE FISHES POSE

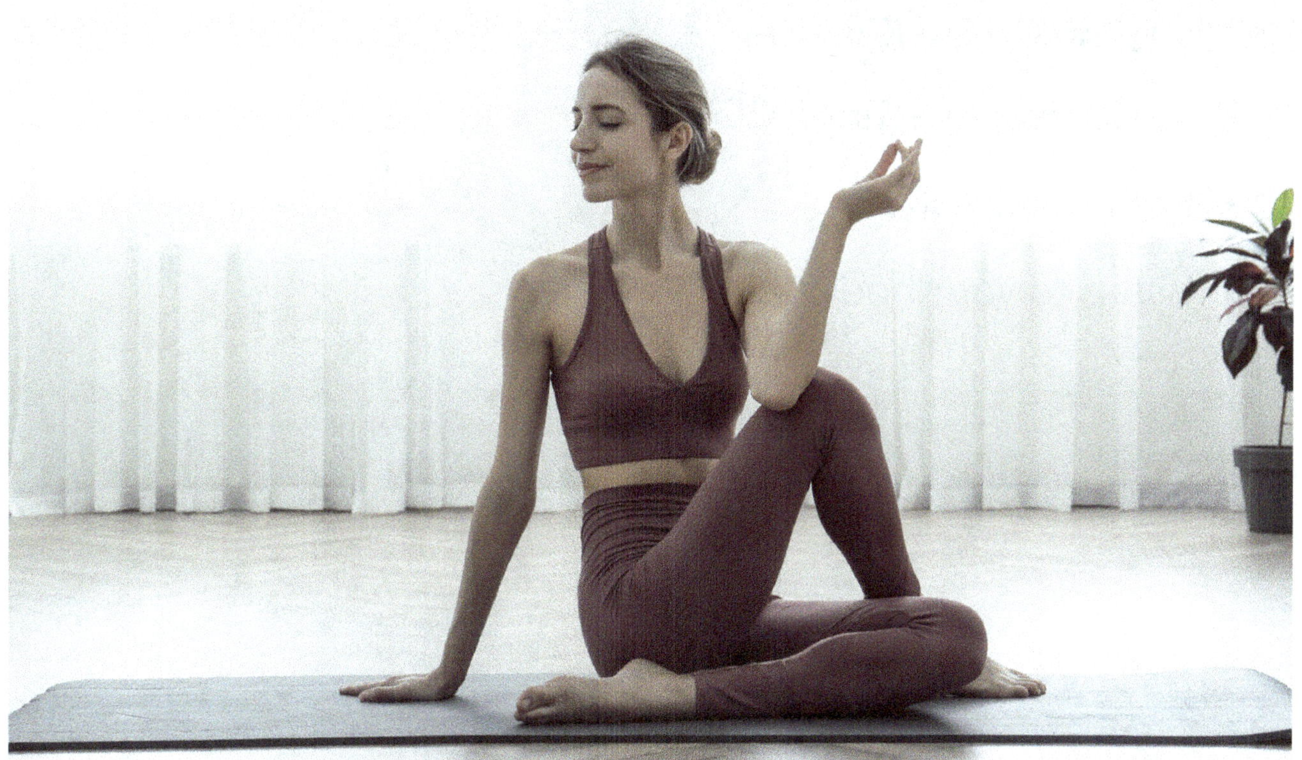

INSTRUCTIONS

- Sit on the mat with your legs extended in front of you.

- Bend your knees and place your feet flat on the mat.

- Cross one leg over the other, planting the foot on the outside of the opposite thigh.

- Inhale, lengthen your spine, and twist towards the bent knee, placing the opposite elbow on the outside of the knee for support.

SAFETY TIPS

- Twist gently from the waist.

- Keep spine tall.

- Engage core slightly.

- Avoid over-twisting.

- Breathe deeply.

- Listen to your body's signals.

RECLINING HAND-TO-BIG-TOE POSE

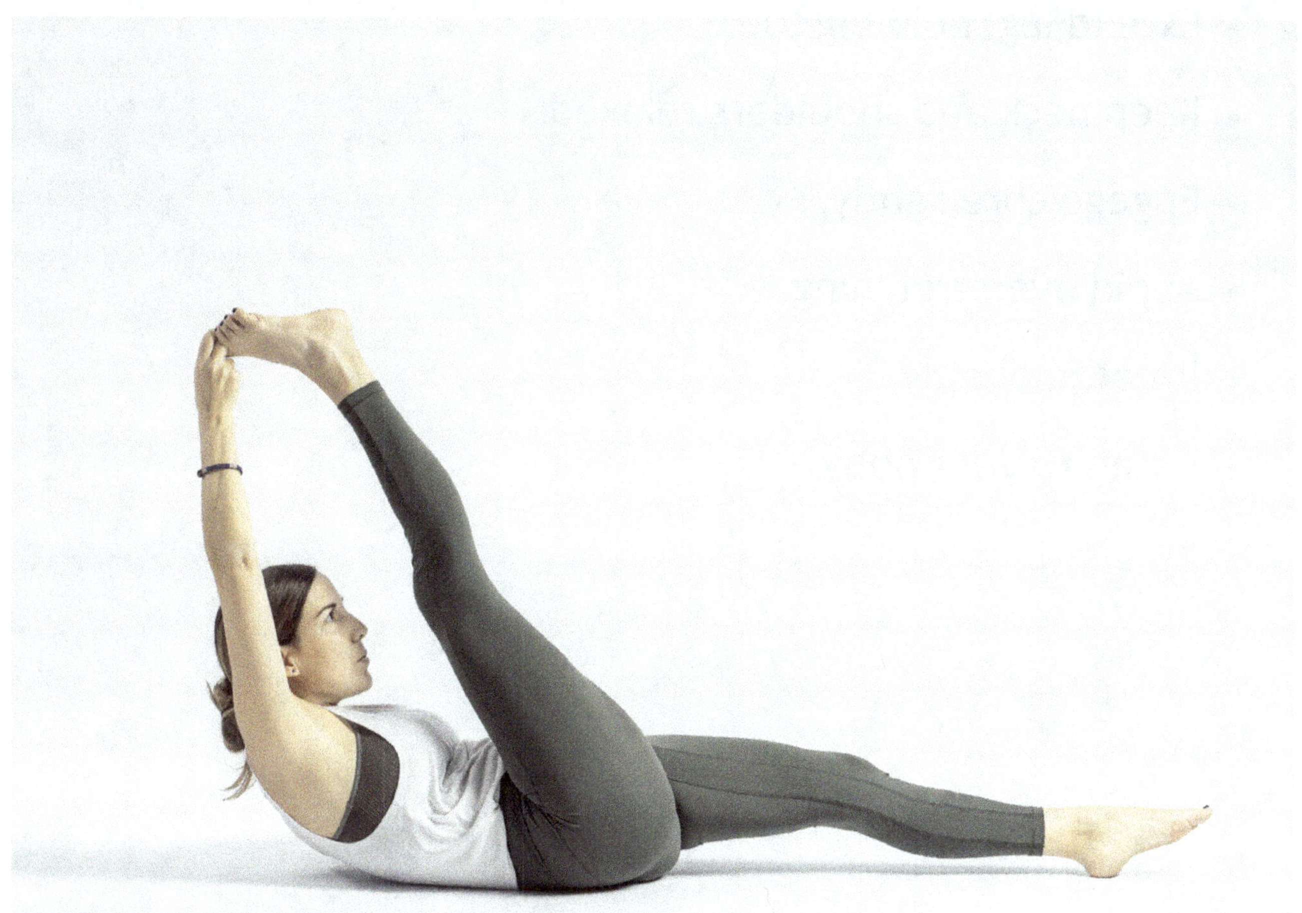

INSTRUCTIONS

- Lie on your back with your legs extended.

- Bend one knee towards your chest and loop a strap around the sole of the foot.

- Straighten the leg towards the ceiling, holding onto the strap with both hands.

- Keep the other leg extended on the mat and your hips grounded.

SAFETY TIPS

- Extend leg, hold big toe.

- Keep neck and shoulders relaxed.

- Engage core lightly.

- Avoid overstretching.

- Breathe deeply.

- Listen to your body.

SUPINE BUTTERFLY POSE

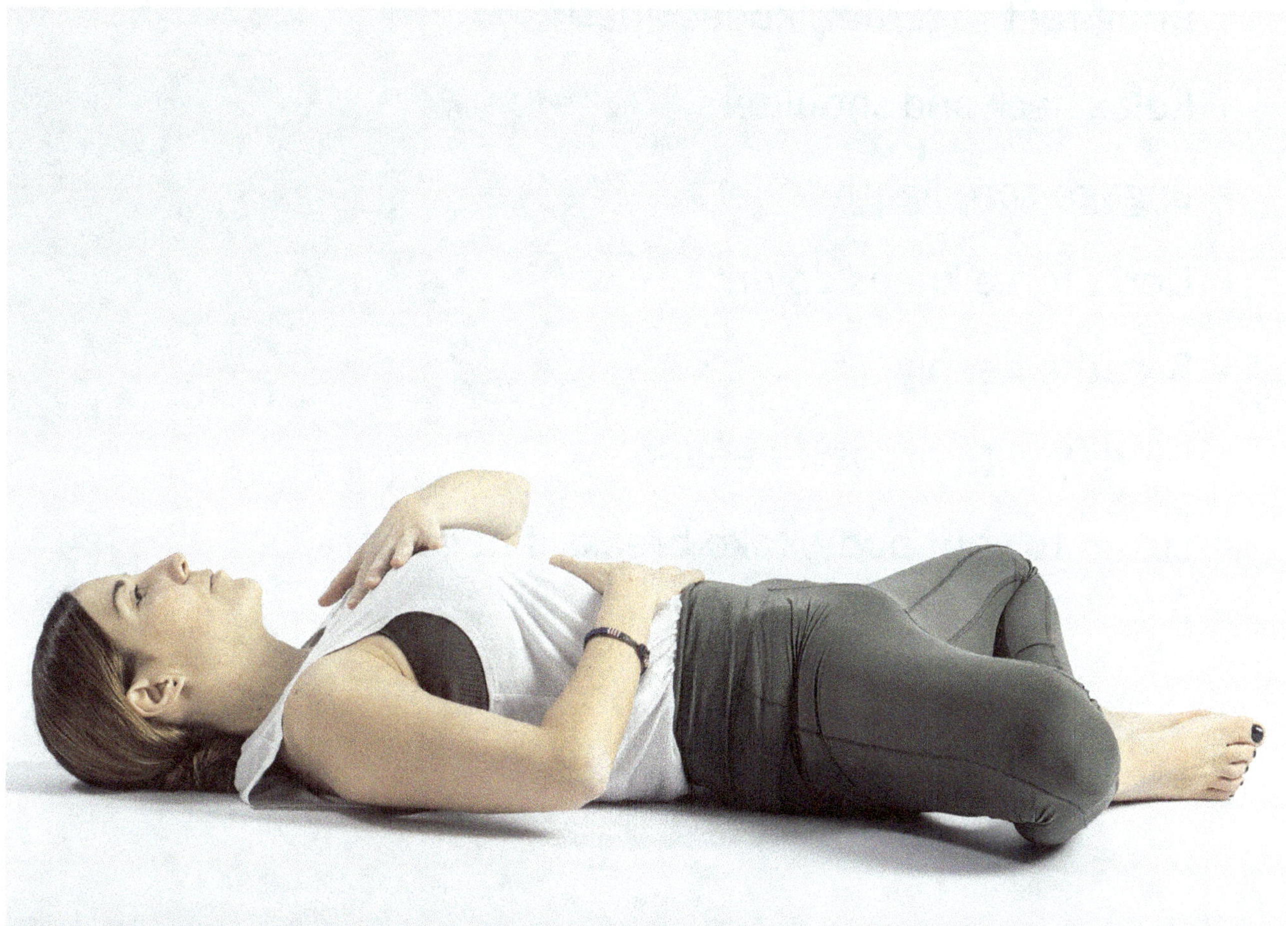

INSTRUCTIONS

- Lie on your back with your knees bent and feet together.

- Let your knees fall open to the sides, bringing the soles of your feet together.

- Allow your hips to open naturally as you relax into the stretch.

SAFETY TIPS

- Bring feet together, knees apart.

- Relax neck and shoulders.

- Engage core lightly.

- Don't force knees down.

- Breathe deeply.

- Modify with props if needed.

- Listen to your body, take breaks if necessary.

STANDING WIDE-LEGGED FORWARD BEND

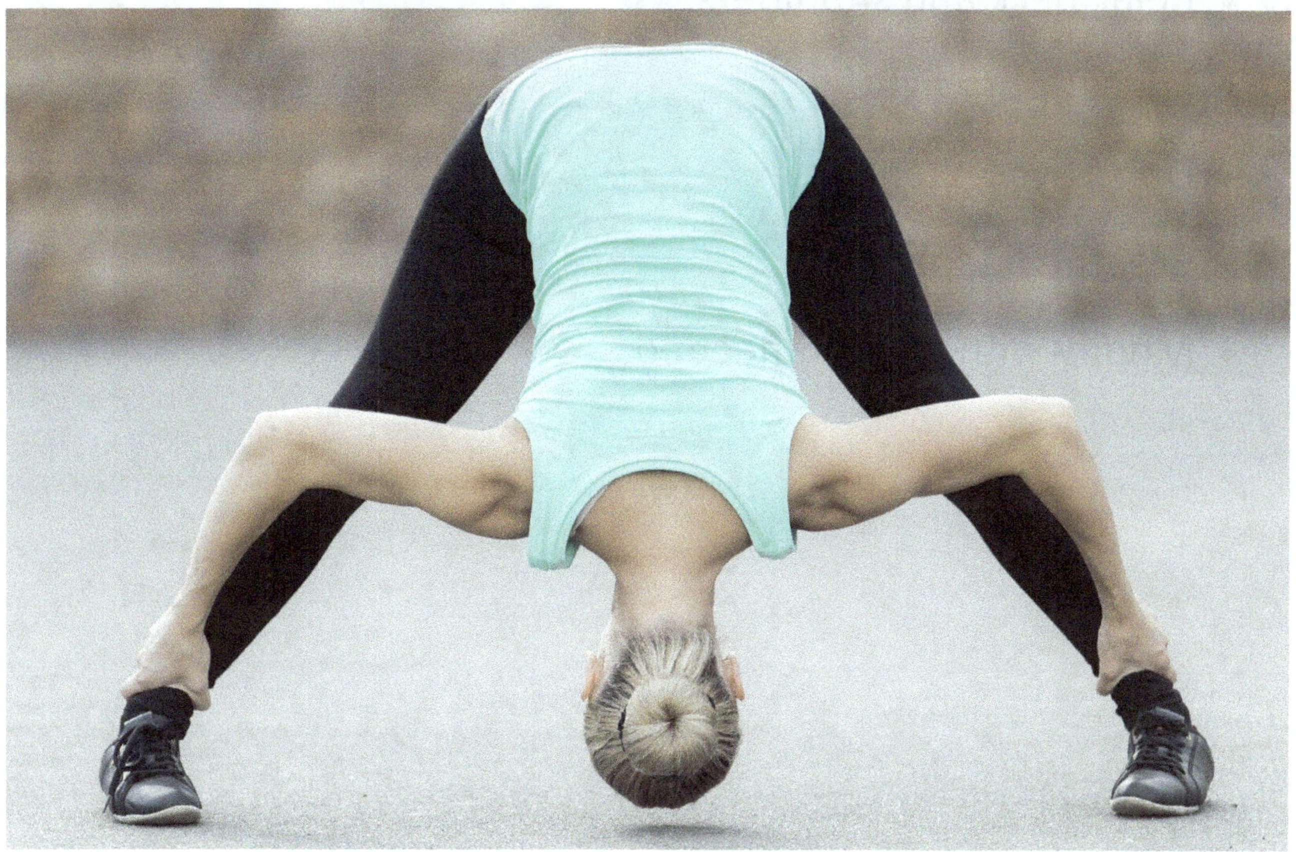

INSTRUCTIONS

- Stand with your feet wider than hip-width apart.

- Interlace your fingers behind your back and straighten your arms.

- Inhale, lengthen your spine, and lift your arms towards the ceiling.

- Exhale, hinge at the hips, and fold forward, bringing your clasped hands overhead.

SAFETY TIPS

- Wide stance, fold forward.

- Relax neck and shoulders.

- Engage core lightly.

- Don't overextend.

- Breathe deeply.

- Modify with props if needed.

CHAIR POSE

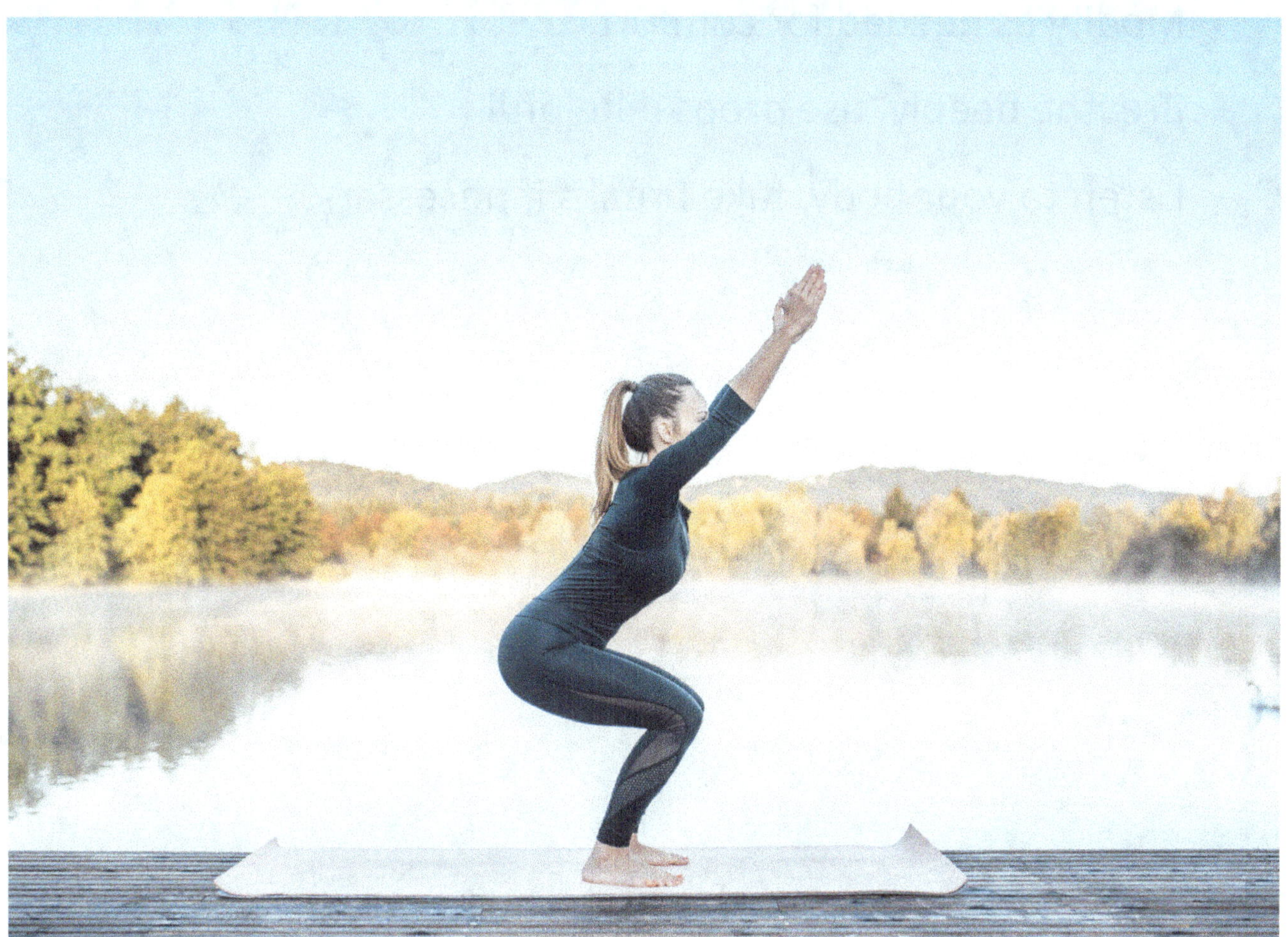

INSTRUCTIONS

- Stand with your feet together or hip-width apart.

- Inhale, raise your arms overhead with palms facing each other.

- Exhale, bend your knees and lower your hips as if sitting back into an imaginary chair.

- Keep your chest lifted and gaze forward.

SAFETY TIPS

- Modify as needed for comfort.

- Breathe deeply, use props if helpful.

- Listen to your body, take breaks if necessary.

CONCLUSION

Through somatic exercises, we not only address the symptoms of back pain but also delve into the underlying causes, unraveling the knots of tension that bind us. With each mindful movement and breath, we forge a deeper connection with our bodies, tapping into their innate wisdom and resilience. As the layers of Sensory Motor Amnesia begin to dissolve, we rediscover the joy of movement, the freedom of expression, and the bliss of being fully present in our bodies. Yet, the journey does not end here. As we integrate somatic exercises into our daily lives, we cultivate a newfound sense of awareness, grace, and empowerment. With patience and dedication, we pave the way for lasting relief, resilience, and radiant health.

So, let us embrace this journey with open hearts and eager spirits, knowing that within the depths of our being lies the power to heal, to thrive, and to flourish.

In the embrace of somatic exercises, may we find not only relief from back pain but also a profound sense of liberation and wholeness.